THE
*Thin*
BOOKS

# THE

# *Thin*

# BOOKS

❋

*Daily Strategies & Meditations
for Fat-Free, Guilt-Free,
Binge-Free Living*

❋

## JEANE EDDY WESTIN

### ▣ HAZELDEN®

Hazelden
Center City, Minnesota 55012-0176

*Library of Congress Cataloging-in-Publication Data*
Westin, Jeane Eddy.
   The thin books : daily strategies and meditations for fat-free, guilt-free, binge-free living / Jeane Eddy Westin.
      p.   cm.
   Based on a revision of the author's The thin book, followed by a full year's worth of meditations from The thin book 2.
   Includes index.
   ISBN 1-56838-108-5
   1. Weight loss—Psychological aspects. I. Westin, Jeane Eddy. Thin book. II. Westin, Jeane Eddy. Thin book 2. III. Title.
RM222.2.W366   1996
613.2'5'019—dc20                                    96-15835
                                                         CIP

*Editor's note*

Hazelden offers a variety of information on chemical dependency and related areas. Our publications do not necessarily represent Hazelden's programs, nor do they officially speak for any Twelve Step organization.

It is wise to consult your physician before beginning any weight-loss or exercise program, especially if you are on medication for chronic medical problems. These medications must be periodically adjusted to reflect weight loss and an improvement in health.

The following organization has generously given permission to use material from a copyrighted work: From *Conjoint Family Therapy.* Used with permission of Avanta: The Virginia Satir Network, 310 Third Avenue NE, Issaquah, WA 98027

To my husband, Gene—
there through thick and thin.

# Contents

**Contents**

## Book II

# Editor's Preface

*The Thin Books* arose out of a recognition that there was a need to both reintroduce and revitalize two of our best-selling books and make them available to a new and expanded audience. *The Thin Book,* a first collection of meditations and exercises, had continued to sell in spite of the trends that had come and gone with respect to weight over the past fifteen years. The principles remained sound, though some of the language and information needed revision. *The Thin Book 2,* a second collection of motivational meditations, had long since gone out of print, and the resources it provided to keep us on track had vanished from the shelves of bookstores.

We decided to create a truly new book, combining the original motivational exercises and prescriptions from the first book and the daily motivational exercises gleaned from the second book. The result is what you now hold, and it holds for you the promise of a healthy life: both the means to understand the hows and whys and what next, and to grant yourself the motivation to continue on the day-to-day quest that is a natural and necessary part of maintaining a healthy body through the means of a healthy mind.

Thus we have *The Thin Books,* not one book but two, not one method but many. On behalf of Hazelden Publishing, we wish you well on your journey.

DAN ODEGARD
*Associate Publisher*

# Acknowledgments

*T*he concept of rewriting *The Thin Book* and *The Thin Book II* and combining them into a more useful format for overeaters did not originate with me. Dan Odegard at Hazelden saw the need, and my editor, Betty Christiansen, made invaluable contributions.

Heartfelt thanks also go to:

- My mother, in memoriam, who loved me no matter what my size and taught me to work hard and to never give up.
- My doctor, Mary Lou Bullen, for her unwavering encouragement, interest, and professional support.
- My friend, Joseph Morrow, Ph.D., who took the mystery out of so many psychological disciplines for me.
- My friends of thirty years, JoAnne, Helen, and Patty, who shared insights about their weight problems, accepted mine, and taught me something about permanence.
- The anonymous woman at a weight group many years ago, who took the hand of a desperate newcomer and said gently, "I know how you feel."
- Robert Siegal, the Healthy Gourmet, who showed me how to cook with no-fat, and whose love of fresh, whole foods was infectious.
- All my friends through the years who, though not overweight, supported my efforts to positively change my relationship with food.

- My extraspecial daughter, Cara, who taught me to find the fun in exercise and has never ceased bolstering my efforts.
- Finally, to all my readers over the years who have shared their personal stories of weight problems and recoveries. I treasure your letters.

# Introduction to Book I

*You are alive.*
*You have a new day.*
*You have another chance.*
*You need your love. Give it.*

*E*very morning I reaffirm these truths to my mirror. But it wasn't always so. Once my waking thoughts were: My life is hopeless! I'm hopeless!—and the day went downhill from there.

You might imagine that I was homeless, destitute, or succumbing to a fatal disease, but you'd be wrong. I had a loving, accepting husband, a darling baby daughter, and career recognition as a writer, which allowed me to pursue creative work that I cared about at home. Sounds like a young woman's dream, doesn't it?

So why did I feel such utter despair? Because my eating was wildly out of control; because I was gaining and losing and gaining again. When the scales hit 272 pounds, my doctor became grim. I remember the solid thunk of the scale's balance bar, followed by his hated words, "morbidly obese," and his threat: "You will never live to raise your child unless you lose weight immediately!" As frightened as I was, I wasn't surprised. For months I had read unspoken questions on the faces of friends, family, and strangers, and on the disgusted face in my own mirror: "How could you let yourself go like that? Where is your willpower?"

But had I let myself go? Hardly. Every day was a struggle, a desperate battle against my compulsion to overeat. I hunted down and tried every diet known on the planet, some good, some terrible—all-fruit, all-protein, high-fat, no-fat, no-sugar, and fasting—always searching for the magical diet that would make me thin. I got hooked on diet pills in the days when doctors routinely prescribed amphetamines for weight control, and went through a painful withdrawal. I risked my health, trying the bulimic behaviors of vomiting and abusing diuretics and laxatives. I risked my life when I submitted to a dangerous intestinal bypass surgery, and then to a reversal operation when I became anemic and my kidneys began to fail.

So where was my lack of willpower? Look at what I'd done to lose weight: I'd starved, swallowed chemicals, and twice submitted to painful, life-threatening surgery. Anyone taking such drastic steps might seem demented, but you'd have to admit they had grit and perseverance.

Why then was I still fat, joyless, and even worse—unhealthy. Headaches, severe nausea, joint pain, low energy, high blood pressure, and borderline diabetes plagued me. What could I do? I had learned that fad diets, pills, and surgery weren't the answers. There seemed to be nothing left.

At that point, I considered giving up—putting my life on hold and accepting my bingeing, unhealthy, unvalued self. The size-acceptance movement had just become vocal, and I agreed that self-esteem shouldn't just come in a size eight. But as hard as I wanted to believe, I wanted to lose weight more. I'd been fat half my life. Was there a way for me to achieve a healthy weight and gain some peace of mind for the second half of my life? I had to try one more time.

And then, out of my despair, came an energizing idea. Instead of waiting for someone to develop a new drug or weight-loss plan to make me thin and well, what if I became proactive? What if I took charge? Could I find within myself something that doctors, surgeons, and diets hadn't given me?

I had been hearing the word *lifestyle* more and more. I liked the idea that "life" could have "style." It seemed to describe freedom from constant food compulsions and dieting. And oh, how I wanted that! But could I create a lifestyle where food had its rightful place? My courage, even my dogged determination hadn't produced any lasting success thus far.

About that time, a local newspaper began using descriptive headlines for its obituaries: "She loved to teach quilting," "She was 'Mama' Morris to the neighborhood," "He fixed broken bikes." I wondered what my claim to fame would be when I died: "She was preoccupied with her diet and full of self-rebuke."

There are times when your spirit is ripe for change and growth. This was one of those times. I'd hit bottom; I was ready to get a life and make the most of it. I decided to begin my new journey by joining a weight-loss group, and being compulsive, I tried several. Each had something to teach me, but I felt most at home with one group that promoted a discipline of rigorous honesty and a step-by-step program of self-discovery and transforming long-held negative attitudes. The group's first and best lesson was that I couldn't take action from a negative stance, only from a positive one. That made sense.

At the group, I met good people—and I met myself. This was the beginning of a life with balance, control, and even style. I lost 111 pounds and dropped eight clothes sizes in fifteen months, a loss that I've maintained for almost twenty years. At first the liberty of a new body was all I wanted. But I soon found that in order to maintain my new weight, I had to go further, dig deeper, learn more. I had to cut to the basics and then, somehow, I had to hold on to those essentials for the rest of my life. Some questions worried me: How had I decided to lose weight and make it stick this time? How had my attitudes changed, and how could I change them further? How could I learn to live well without my buffer of fat?

As a writer, I've found that one of the most powerful paths to self-discovery is to write down and confront what you think. Amazing truths leap out of your subconscious and onto paper. Things make sense for the first time. The journal I kept during my discovery process became the basis for *The Thin Books*. Each day's journal entry became part of my personal blueprint, reinforcing the truths I'd found within myself, the truths that others had shared with me, and the truths that overeating had always kept me from confronting.

It was a wonderful time. My journal pages revealed not just a woman with excess weight, not just someone with problems, but a complete person, imperfect, but with many qualities. This was someone I liked a lot, someone I wanted for a friend. After half a lifetime, I was no longer at war with myself.

As I shed negative attitudes, I gained a mission: I wanted to help others achieve a healthy weight, to start hitting positive notes, and to stop hitting on themselves.

*The Thin Books,* filled with positive insights, tips, and techniques, will help you deal with food control, find alternatives to the old "shame and blame" game, discover a new way to live more effectively, and achieve a self-understanding which makes self-esteem possible.

But *The Thin Books* gives you more than positive tips, insights, and self-understanding—it helps you grow into a winning attitude. Simply put, *The Thin Books* will help you "be" and then "do," and you must "do" before you can "have."

And finally, *The Thin Books* will allow you to see yourself as you really are—a uniquely magnificent individual who can say "Yes!" to every new day. Remember this: Living well is all about attitude.

A final word: use this book hard—underline passages, write in the margins, and make it your own journal of discovery.

# CHAPTER 1

# Changing Your Life

## Getting Started

*Y*ou've already started. When you picked up this book and began to read, you got on your mark. Now you're ready, set to run the rest of the way, and you want to win. You're ready to change your life.

Something brought you to this point. Maybe you're in the midst of a crisis, maybe you're asking yourself searching questions and looking everywhere for answers, or perhaps you're at a physical and spiritual crossroads. Whatever your situation, if you're willing to reevaluate your attitudes and rid yourself of all the eating cover-ups, you're right on track. This is your wake-up call.

Nobody claims that turning your life around will be easy or fast, and you wouldn't believe them if they did. Changing from negative to positive attitudes is an enormous challenge. Gaining daily mastery over the way you use food will take all you've already got. But you've got all it will take.

How, exactly, do you activate your own inner resources?

Start with this first section of *The Thin Books*. It will help you establish an effective new emotional base of resolution, motivation, and commitment. From this foundation, you'll be ready to move confidently forward to greater challenges. The trick to winning is to stay motivated.

One of the best ways to stay motivated is to keep your spirit soaring by casting off negative experiences and intensifying positive ones. If your spirits rise, your weight falls. It sounds simple, but most truth is just that uncomplicated.

Frankly, you have to guard your positive attitude like Fort Knox. Negativity is everywhere, and it's a diet-killer. Steer clear of thoughts or people who say, "You tried diets before and gained it all back," or, "Hey, it's in your genes." So what if you've gained and lost weight? Who hasn't? And science may or may not find a fat gene someday. So what? You're here now and you want to live today. Don't let anyone pull you down.

Rather, seek out affirming people—friends and family or a group—who will listen and support you when you need help. Next, gather in all your positive experiences. Know which ones motivate you toward your goal. Think about all of your positive life experiences, times when you felt intensely good about yourself, when you liked what you saw in your mirror. Call those positive feelings back whenever you need them, and make them work for you again.

There's something else for you to add to the mix as you begin: a special commitment. Here, you need to take a page from corporate business. Ninety percent of all major companies in America have what is called a mission statement. It's a surefire way for successful companies to state a vision for future success.

You can adopt this effective tool to motivate yourself every day. Take five minutes right now and come up with your own official mission statement. Make it simple, affirmative, and inspiring. Here's one that works well:

> *My mission is a commitment to lose weight, maintain a healthy body, and seek a life that affords me the chance to exercise my talents—sooner rather than later.*

You may want to include a specific weight or life goal; it's up to you. Whatever your mission, write it down and post it in a place where you'll see it several times a day. Go ahead and frame your mission statement; it shows your serious intent and keeps you focused.

Remember, the only limits are those you impose on yourself. Every day you learn something is an adventure. Today you can reach out for more life than you have now, and tomorrow reach out again. Yes, you've tried before. But this time you're not just *trying,* you're *doing.* And, as you progress, you'll be amazed with what you can accomplish.

It's your life. Get ready to live it!

## Resolution

You know what day this is. It's diet resolution day. Whether you're ten pounds or two hundred pounds overweight, whether this is Monday or New Year's Day, today is D-day for your healthier eating plan, on which you will lose the weight you want and come to love your body.

What are you promising yourself and anyone else who might be listening? *"This time, I'm going to lose weight, never to be fat again."* What a bright future those words envision. How much hope they contain. But how often in the past have they lost their meaning all too soon?

Well, get ready for the surprise of your life. This time, your promise is not just so many brave words flung defiantly at the calendar. Each day you have another chance to get on a weight-losing diet that really works. What miracle diet is this? Simply the one you are on today.

Because every day is today. The high-calorie food you ate yesterday (and feel guilty about) and the food you might eat tomorrow (and fear) don't count. What *does* count is what you eat this day and how you feel about it. This is the day you can become who you really are—empowered and energized.

For the moment, do not worry about how many pounds you must lose or how long it will take you to lose them. You must live through the days, weeks, and months whether you are losing weight or not. Focus instead on how you will live them—overwhelmed by diet disaster or successfully following your weight-losing program one day at a time. Say it out loud: *"This is the year I'm going to lose weight, never to be fat again."*

### Get on Your Mark

Like Scarlett O'Hara in *Gone with the Wind,* an overeater's philosophy of life often is "I won't worry about that today; I'll worry about that tomorrow." Of course, in a way, that's right. Tomorrow *is* another day. But what's wrong with right now?

Too often for us, tomorrow never comes. There are too many tomorrows, too many jokes about the fat person who says, "I'm starting my diet next Monday." Delaying tactics can be helpful in managing anger, but counting to ten before you start a life without excess food is a big mistake.

*Do it now!* When you delay, desire dies. If you truly want to live a life that isn't dominated by what you're going to eat next, get started now. If you are sick and tired of your dependency on certain foods, take immediate action.

If you feel overwhelmed by obstacles, focus on possibilities instead: You will be able to target a lower, healthier weight and lighten your emotional load as well. You will gain self-respect, a body you'll like to live in, and an alertness that will no longer be dulled by the physical assault of too many calories. These are the positive promises you can give yourself today. Delaying only gives you another twenty-four hours of confusion and pain.

And when you delay, what you're really postponing is life. You may not die if you don't lose excess weight, but you won't live—*really* live—either.

You can fill your life with rich meaning, with choices. Begin by making this important first choice: commit yourself to eating the proper foods in the proper balance, increasing your exercise, and growing in at least one area of your emotional life. Do you want to turn your life around, lose your excess weight, and live with dignity? If so, commit yourself to change.

Four years ago, Anna had her first baby. She's still wearing the same maternity clothes today. "I'm too embarrassed to buy new clothes," she confesses. "When I walk into a store, I can sense the sales consultant eyeing me with disgust. I'm afraid she'll find something hideous and tell me I'd better grab it because it's all she has in my size."

Anna's response always has been to go home and eat, avoiding mirrors, hiding from her body, running from herself. But now she says, "When I have the courage to look in my mirror, I *know* I've got to lose weight. I've *got* to!" This story, admitted tearfully at a diet-group meeting, is the first evidence that Anna is willing to come out of hiding.

## Motivation

Food is the great cover-up. For Anna and many of us, fat takes us out of the mainstream of life and gives us a ready-made excuse to cut off involvement with the rest of the world. We all know the trap of too many pounds—fat can create enormous physical and emotional barriers. Of the two, the emotional barrier is the higher.

But when you begin to think that there *is* hope and you *can* lose weight, then you begin to stop hiding from yourself and others. You become motivated to let your creative mind get to work and you begin to see yourself as a capable, positive, and worthwhile person. This is the key that opens the door to your new life.

Unfortunately, most diet programs assume this motivation is *already* there. Just getting psyched up to begin another run for the prize can be our biggest obstacle. Long-time dieters, like distance runners, don't have too much trouble starting, if they could only get to the starting block.

### Get Set

Many times that all-important motivation comes in a *moment of recognition,* a moment when you realize you cannot postpone your life any longer. You wake up one morning saying: "I've had it with living this way. I'm going to change, *now.*" You decide with great determination that you will not postpone; you will not wait until after the next snack or even until tomorrow. You are overcome by a strong, irresistible urge to start *immediately.*

You can help bring about this moment of recognition by taking two important steps: admitting you need to lose weight and then accepting that fact. Neither is easy, and motivation may not come overnight. But these two steps provide an important foundation for making change happen.

1. *Admission.* It seems unnecessary to tell overweight people that the first step in self-motivation is an admission that they have problems with food. And yet, if it weren't necessary, why would members of some weight-loss groups preface their talks with, "Hi, my name is Mary, and I'm a compulsive overeater"? The reason for the admission is simple. We are notorious self-deceivers. How often have we characterized our extra poundage as baby fat, big bones, gland problems, or a host of other euphemisms? Most of us call ourselves anything but fat. But admitting that we are fat is the first step toward self-honesty, without which there can be no motivation.

2. *Acceptance.* Admitting and accepting are two different things and, of the two, accepting is harder. If you are someone who says, "Yes, I'm fat," and continues overeating and gaining weight, then you're not accepting yourself as you really are. The act of acceptance implies action. When you accept the reality of your body, you will be ready for your own moment of recognition, a moment that will take you to the starting block of your race for a healthier body, a happier outlook, and an inner peace. You will have made the choice to make a change.

When you make this choice to do something positive with your life, your motivation level is high. The next step is to target a goal and begin moving toward it, one day at a time.

Unless our motivation is high, we invariably slip and fall off even the healthiest eating plan. Then what do we say? "It didn't work." "It made me too uncomfortable." Typically, we relied on diet alone to make us slender, rather than blending an eating plan with a new set of positive attitudes and a generally healthier lifestyle.

Is your desire to lose weight and change your life stronger than your desire for food? That is the question, and only you can answer it. If you've had enough—if you feel you've suffered enough—you are ready.

This motivation, this deep desire to change, isn't just something you need for a few minutes when beginning a new way of eating. It is a lifelong feeling kept alive by the memory of the food-centered life you are leaving behind. Your mind's desire, the thin, healthy you, is not mere daydreaming. It is the way you really see yourself. It is your own blueprint for change.

## Commitment

Carlos Castaneda wrote, "When a man [or woman] decides to do something he [or she] must go all the way."

The people who successfully keep their excess weight off seem to be people who do just that—go all the way. "My whole life depends on not overeating," said one person in a special meeting for maintaining weight. "Nothing in the world can make me overeat. I have promised myself I won't do it. And I won't break my promise to myself. I feel that I have given up my right to overeat, and that decision, once made, is final."

Prepare to go all the way, as if your whole life depended on it. It does. Don't let the child in you say, "I probably won't be able to do it." You don't need a cushion against failure that allows you to later say, "There, I knew I couldn't do it." A half-commitment that says grudgingly, "Okay, I'll try," isn't enough either. It is a response motivated by fear of failure.

Make a full-fledged commitment to going all the way with your healthy eating plan. Say, like the successful maintainer, "Nothing in the world can make me overeat."

*Go!*

There are five actions you'll need to take to help make this new master plan a reality. Don't worry about having to develop new qualities or skills; the resources needed to take these actions are already part of your character—you just have to tap into them:

1. *Take risks.* One of the reasons why we give up on our ability to lose weight before really giving it a try is that we dare not risk failure. Failure to lose weight has always devastated us. As we grow older, we learn to protect ourselves from hurt in advance; thereby we sacrifice our desire for emotional growth and a slimmer body in exchange for security. Once you discover that security is not possible where there is no control over food, then you will stop playing it so safe.

2. *Get ready to go it alone.* Others may not always be there for you when you need them. "I have a sponsor, many friends, and a supportive family," said one diet club member, "and still I am alone when I confront the Oreos." When it comes down to it, you are your most reliable source of strength.

3. *Make a commitment.* Don't allow anything to sidetrack you from your commitment to a healthier, happier life.

4. *Believe you can do it.* If you believe in yourself, you can accept your "downs" as well as your "ups," and you will have *real* pride in your ability to change your life. When you truly believe you can lose weight, maintain a healthy weight, and restructure your attitudes for happiness, you won't ever have to put up the "false front" of overeating again.

5. *Accept change.* You have mature, consistent values that will help you make it through change without overeating.

Now that you know what's needed to change your life, begin. Call up the skills necessary to take these five actions, skills which you have always possessed but which have been lying dormant. Start building your new life and begin living it today.

You might feel overwhelmed at the number of ways you want to change your life and the time and patience required to make those changes happen. Don't try to take on too much too soon. Take one problem at a time. You may have many problems, but start on your weight problem first. We kid ourselves when we think we can postpone losing weight until every other problem in our lives is resolved. Being overweight is the problem that has you on your knees right now. After you begin to lose pounds, you can tackle your other troubles, one at a time, as you're ready. Surprisingly, other problems sometimes don't look like problems when we remove the veil of overeating.

Working toward a thin, healthy body is worth every effort. This will be a time when you are vitally alive, awake, and enthusiastic. It will be the best time of your life.

# CHAPTER 2

# Positive Thinking

## Changing Your Attitudes about Yourself

*I*s your inner voice filled with *can'ts, wouldn'ts, shouldn'ts, couldn'ts?* If these are the words you hear when you tune in to yourself, fasten your seatbelt, it's going to be a bumpy life. Such unhealthy attitudes only sabotage you. Successful people, the people who strive for and maintain a slender, healthy body, hear "I can" messages. They have developed the habit of thinking positively.

Unsuccessful people adopt negative attitudes to protect themselves from failure. Later they can shrug and say, "Well, I knew I wouldn't make it; at least I was right about that!" But how can negative self-fulfilling prophecies possibly produce a slender, healthy body, or self-esteem and well-being? They can produce nothing but certain failure.

With a positive outlook, you won't need such false protection. You can risk making a mistake, because you can learn from it and then let it go.

Take a look at how positive people live. Healthy thinkers, people who feel they deserve the good life, say: "Hey, nobody's perfect. What did I do right and how can I build on it to do even better?" Adopting this attitude will allow you to stop tearing yourself down and

**17**

start building yourself up to be the person you always wanted to be. It's about time to become emotionally responsible and develop healthy attitudes. You have to do this for yourself—no one else will do it for you.

Sometimes we overeaters are all-or-nothing people; we can't accept less than our idea of exaggerated perfection. However, this type of thinking is exactly what has led us to fall off our weight-losing diet plans in the past. To succeed this time, we'll need to change our negative, self-defeating attitude to a positive, self-affirming one. We'll have to work at cultivating this positive way of thinking one day at a time, in ordinary situations. For example, if you're ever disappointed by the reading on your bathroom scale, try to be a nurturing friend to yourself, acknowledging your best efforts realistically, instead of being negative about being a little less than best.

Negative, cruel self-criticism is a form of hate, an inability to look lovingly and gently at yourself and your situation. Love yourself just as you are today. Does such self-love sound selfish or impossible because you're not perfect? Accepting a loving self is not the same as having a big ego. Like the old song says, life without love "ain't no life at all." With love of self, you will be able to love others and to love success; love of self will help free you of food dependence and put you into the thinner body you desire.

As you begin to use food in healthier ways, you may feel emotionally deprived. That's natural. Remember, you have used food to control feelings of anger, boredom, fear, and unhappiness; you used food for comfort and to relieve tension. It didn't work—food didn't block the feelings, and you gained weight.

But you are about to have a transforming experience.

So give yourself time for new, healthy habits and self-affirming attitudes to take hold. You are no longer a slave to the past; your positive mind is in charge today.

Just for this single day, try to focus on your best qualities, not on your problem. Don't be critical; just be honest. Take five minutes right now to remember times when you were loving, open, trusting, self-respectful, patient, or caring.

Do you see what just happened? For the past five positive minutes, you have been out of your problem, you have not craved unhealthy food, and you have not beat on yourself over your weight or shortcomings, real or imagined. Isn't that a stunning recognition?

This new, healthier focus will lead you to actively and repeatedly encourage success. But it only works when you work it. It's an *active* partnership.

Think of yourself as a scriptwriter, writing a script for your own life. You may believe your script was already written by your parents, by your genetic makeup, or by any number of other people. And you may think you have no control over the outcome. Like our Puritan forefathers, you may believe in the concept of predestination. But the idea that everything is preordained would mean that nobody has a chance to change, so why bother trying?

A "what's-the-use" attitude can't build your new, thin, successful life. If you think you've been handed a lousy script, rewrite it. Eliminate whatever hinders you. Start by eliminating negative (or fat) thinking—it hasn't worked for you thus far.

When you're writing your script remember one thing: Hollywood producers rarely buy a story with an unhappy ending; they know that audiences don't like gloom and doom. So why try to sell a bleak life script to yourself? Write a happy ending to your life story. Take positive charge of your food desires and unhealthy thinking habits; begin seeing the possibilities ahead and not the problems.

In the following pages, you'll find specific thinking skills you can learn and information on how and when to use them to write your happy ending. Remember, no one knows you better than you do, and no one can better personalize a script for your success.

## It Starts with You

In Chapter 1, "Changing Your Life," you determined that you were ready to start preparing for lifelong diet success right *now*. Whether you are sixteen or forty or sixty-five, it starts right now. And starts with you—with your own powerful, positive image. This is basic to success because such an image gives you *permission* to learn and to change.

You must have noticed that some people lose their excess weight while others only lose their way and sink into a pit of hopelessness. Have you ever passed off successful weight loss to luck, superior intelligence, education, or money? These are actually insignificant factors. Attitudes for success are what make the real difference.

First and foremost, successful people believe that *their dreams can come true.* They consider nothing impossible and have a reservoir of faith in themselves.

Second, *they are capable of quick adaptation.* They intuitively understand that they can't stand still, that life moves on every day, taking them with it.

In addition, while they may have fear, successful people don't let fear stop them. *They work through problems* in spite of every difficulty. They act as if they have courage whether they feel courageous or not.

Finally, *they give each goal along their way enough time*

*to happen.* We compulsive eaters are impatient people; we want to take off weight *right now.* Those of us who lose weight successfully realize that every day is important to the learning, growing process, and that we'll need all these days to be ready to live the thin life.

Ask yourself if you fit this picture of success. Do you believe your dream can come true? Are you willing to move forward a little each day? Can you work through problems without giving up? Are you able to give each goal enough time to transpire? If you don't fit this picture now, don't give up—you can learn. This is the very image of a positive, creative thinker, the person who makes dreams come true.

Attitude alone will not ensure weight loss. However, the combination of a positive attitude with knowledge and the ability to act on that knowledge is a surefire recipe for success: successful people develop the knowledge that overeating is harmful to their health and self-esteem. Second, they believe that quitting overeating is the paramount experience in their lives. Third, they turn their knowledge and attitude into permanent behavior changes that ensure their continuing success.

The difference between these people and those who do not accomplish their goals is a simple matter of positive programming. When you program your mind to reflect a healthy self-image, you can think better, perform better, and feel better.

### Accentuate the Positive

Many years ago, songwriter Johnny Mercer wrote a hit song called "Accentuate the Positive," which could easily become the anthem of overeaters everywhere. Mercer's upbeat tune suggested that people "latch on to the affirmative, eliminate the negative."

Despite Mercer's good advice, many people accentuate

the negative instead. And it's no wonder. Overweight people in American society are bombarded with visual messages that reinforce a negative self-image. For example, television tells us, in so many words and pictures, that we are not physically attractive if we are not the superthin ideal. If you're overweight in this "thin" world, you can't avoid picking up attitudes critical of overweight people in general and about yourself in particular. You read that a worker is discharged because of obesity; this underscores the idea that fat people are lazy and can't keep up. You turn on your television and the thin bodies of celebrities remind you that you really shouldn't "let yourself go."

Influenced in part by messages such as these, some of us believe that thinness and self-worth are one and the same. They are not. We do want healthy bodies that look and feel good, but weight has nothing to do with our value as human beings.

Negative thinking suggests that, if we are overweight, we deserve unhappiness. The slightest cutting remark poisons our day and affirms our *own* bad opinion of ourselves. Nothing is more deadly than negative thinking. It saps energy, makes us unpleasant companions, and plays havoc with the development of sensible eating habits.

*Beating the Enemy Within*

"There is a silent, subconscious internal conversation taking place within our minds," says psychologist and author Dr. Jerry Schmidt. "This conversation actually determines how we feel about what is taking place in the external world." Often, says the doctor, this inner conversation is so negative it can immobilize us. Daily effort can bring negativity under control.

It's important for dieters not to let negative thoughts

take root. For instance, if you really begin to believe you can't stand your new, healthier way of eating, you can soon convince yourself that you shouldn't be dieting in the first place. If you believe that you must be happy *all* the time, thinking something is wrong with you if you aren't, you are leaving the way open for compensatory eating, for thinking your sorrows can be soothed with food.

Ridding yourself of destructive negative thinking doesn't happen overnight. It takes time like anything else worthwhile, but with persistence, you can learn one day at a time.

The first step to becoming a positive thinker is to get rid of all preconditioned negative thinking. When you were a child, you believed the concepts fed to you by adults. But you are no longer a child to be led like a lamb, prey to the misconceptions and misleading messages that abound in today's society. If negative thinking is destroying your life, then begin to use your mind's potential to change things.

For example, you may have been told, "You're just a fat slob and there's nothing you can do about it." This and other negative messages, attitudes given to you by others, can cause you untold misery. Sadly enough, long after the old influences are gone, your preconditioned negative thinking goes right on controlling your actions, so that every day your life becomes what you think.

If you allow your negative thoughts and emotions to dominate you, you'll become a frustrated pessimist, and most likely stay fat. If you allow negativity to promote disharmony within your thinking, you will find yourself constantly out of step with reality.

On the other hand, if you allow your personality and developing master plan of healthy living to be guided by positive thoughts, your enthusiasm will help keep you on your chosen path.

### The Power of Choice

Now it's time to be aware of your own power and let go of negativity. Start immediately by identifying new attitudes you want to develop. Counter worry with faith, suspicion with trust, sorrow with joy, resignation with determination, gloom with cheer, anxiety with security, hostility with friendliness, and guilt with forgiveness.

For every negative emotion there is an opposite positive emotion. You have a choice. You choose your own emotional makeup. Philosopher William James gave this advice for uncovering the positive treasure of your mind: "Seek out the particular mental . . . attitude in which [makes you feel] most deeply and intensely active and alive. At such moments there is a voice inside which speaks and says: 'This is the real me!'"

You are acquiring a new, empowered inner voice. Listen to it. You can't stop it. Bingeing can't stop it. Overeating only quiets your inner voice for a moment, and then it reappears stronger than ever. Allow this positive voice inside you to become a conscious action. Listen to the "real you," and act on what you hear.

Like a marble, you are waiting for the sculptor's hand to free the real you by chipping away the excess stone. But this time you are both marble and artist. You will free yourself by your own healthy attitudes. When you have established your true identity, when you have listened to your supportive inner voice, your life will move in a new direction. Doors that were closed will open. Possibilities will become realities.

Best of all, you will have control over a physical function called eating—a small part of living that nearly ruined your life.

Listen to the encouraging inner voice that tells you who you really are. Seek out the attitude that makes you feel alive. Trust it. You *do* deserve your best.

## Choose to Win

Nobody ever said that losing weight and maintaining a healthy, thin body would be easy. This is clearly the most important battle you are ever likely to fight.

Sometimes our problem looms so large on the scale, we become overwhelmed. Those excess pounds, whether twenty or one hundred, appear to be insurmountable. Our future seems dim indeed, if it means more of the same roller-coaster binge-diet way of life. But you are not a captive passenger on this ride. Now you have something to say about what happens in your life. *Now you have control.*

The philosopher Kahlil Gibran said: "Your daily life is your temple and your religion. Whenever you enter into it take with you your all." Have you entered your life today with all your resolve and all your will, or are you floundering with only half your mental resources? Are you willing to let each day be your "religion," or are you devoid of any faith in yourself? Do you see how self-doubt interferes with living?

Just below your conscious mind lies destructive old mind-sets etched in stone. They tell you that you "don't stand a chance," that you "always fail so go ahead and give up." But your creative mind can produce positive images just as easily as negative ones. You need only give it positive input. In your mind's eye, see yourself eating healthfully and getting thinner and more content each day. See your family and friends, even strangers, accepting your new image. See yourself as a self-responsible person for whom pity in any form is absolutely unnecessary. See yourself as a person who functions well on every level. Act, don't react.

*Where There's a Will . . .*

An eastern philosopher suggests we say to ourselves: "I will be what I will to be. I will do what I will to do."

Here is the most positive affirmation of your mind's power. This statement contains complete positive energy. There is no hesitation, no limiting phrase, no "maybe."

We overeaters fill our lives with *maybes, buts,* and *sometimes.* We approach life too tentatively. But saying, "I will be what I will to be, I will do what I will to do," bestows boldness on us. It gives us inner strength and control.

Instead of applying the tentative word *maybe* to your goals, try using the positive word *will.* You will find that the force of this word will stabilize your thinking and give you new hope.

As you are learning, the power of a positive thought is very strong. It can awaken intense feelings, especially when you repeat it again and again. Each repetition will become a new imprint on your conscious mind, giving you the power you need when you need it.

Your strong, creative thoughts and a commitment to them will help you get to know the great inner person you really are. You will be what you will to be; you will do what you will to do. You have made that decision, a decision to do something about your weight and your health.

If you're at a loss as to what decisions you can act upon today, try one of these:

1. *Decide* that you can't "have your cake and eat it too." Withstand one temptation today.

2. *Decide* that today you will start the rest of your life. Take one action to reflect that.

3. *Decide* that your best investment is in yourself. Give yourself one nonfood-related treat today.

4. *Decide* that with a positive, healthy attitude you

can't help but win. Make a list of positive statements about yourself and reflect on them.

5. *Decide* that a new pattern of positive action will result from your new pattern of thinking. List the positive actions you've taken already today.

6. *Decide* to expand your capacity to absorb more and more positive thoughts. What positive attributes can you find in the people around you?

7. *Decide* to accept no more excuses for overeating. Stop yourself when you find yourself justifying an extra bite today.

8. *Decide* that nothing free is worth having, and that you will not be able to get by with a minimum effort. Don't opt for the easy—but less effective—solution to a problem today.

9. *Decide* that you must keep busy. Make a list of activities to do when boredom—and the subsequent urge to eat—sets in.

10. *Decide* to choose to live today slender and healthy. Write a statement reflecting this choice, and read it often today.

You are capable of making good decisions and good choices for your new, thin life. You are learning ways to incorporate them into action.

*Flex Your Positive Muscles*

Combating negativism is a dieter's first line of defense in the battle for a thin, healthy body. Therefore, it is important to begin each day by thinking of all the things *right* about you. As was suggested in the preceding list, it's a good idea to actually put them on paper so you can *see* them. Later you may only need to make a mental list. But do make a list, review it often, and as you grow thinner, keep adding new, positive attributes to it. Don't let one negative image creep in.

Why is it so important to flex your positive muscles like this? In order to diet victoriously you must first feel good about yourself—good enough to go to work for yourself—not for anyone else. It may sound selfish, but victors in the fight against fat are generally people who want to lose weight for themselves. There's nothing wrong with that—self-interest is a powerful motivator.

There are a number of tools we can use to look at ourselves objectively and to record the good things we find. Making a list is one. Another is keeping a "pleasure diary," in which you write down all your daily activities as they occur and decide on the spot whether they constitute an accomplishment. Quite often, people who have formerly been very hard on themselves will discover that they do a number of things quite well. Then it becomes increasingly more difficult to make sweeping statements such as, "I can never do anything right."

Real and lasting success consists of a series of little daily victories. Listing your daily victories, no matter how small they are, can help you see this. These victories can include such seemingly trivial things as being patient with a neighbor who asks too many questions about your weight, not eating compulsively, laughing, or congratulating yourself on a two-pound loss.

It will not take too many days before you discover that you are having more pleasant experiences than you ever realized. You will soon note that your low moods are directly related to negative thinking and that your pleasure diary helps you change from being a pessimist to being an optimist. After all, it is difficult to continue thinking negatively when you have proof of accomplishment right there in writing.

Take a close look at your lists and your diary; read over all the little victories and achievements of your day. You'll find there are more of them than you ever imagined.

*The Chocolate Factory Syndrome*

In order to be a winner in the "positive game," we must let positive forces permeate our entire lives. We must select positive stimuli and block negative stimuli which come to us through many channels. *Just as you wouldn't expose your body to the temptations of working in a chocolate factory, you shouldn't expose your mind to similarly negative forces.*

Quickly evaluate the negative influences in your life. Can you improve in any of the following areas?

1. *Reading materials:* Does the material you choose stimulate positive emotions? Do you read popular magazines filled with images of superthin models, or do you choose to read magazines and books that promote positive, healthful ways of eating and living?

2. *Entertainment, such as film or television:* Do the movies and programs you choose have positive messages?

3. *Friends:* Are your friends positive-minded and supportive?

4. *Language:* Do you hear yourself saying, "What's the use?" If you voice such defeatism, you give your negative side added power to control you. On the other hand, if your speech is positive and upbeat—"I'm getting thinner and stronger every day"—you add a powerful ally in your march toward your goal.

As you can see, you have to guard your positive self from negative people and outside sources, but particularly from your sabotaging self.

Why is such a mental exercise necessary? Generally, overweight people have had a rough time of it. Many of us have been told we were self-indulgent, lacking in willpower, and, heaven forbid, even immoral! And that's just what *others* have called us. We have called ourselves much worse in the depth of our despair.

Consequently, some of us have a very low opinion of ourselves as human beings.

If there is any group of people that needs to look on the bright side, it's overweight people. And yet, despite the apparent need, some dieters cannot seem to find much that is good to say about themselves. If you can't find much good in yourself, start giving your positive self as much exercise as you used to give your negative self.

To switch your subconscious pattern from negative to positive you will need to mold new ideas into your mental processes. You can do this with affirmation, by combining words and mind pictures. Begin by seeing yourself with new, more tolerant eyes. Treat yourself like you'd treat a special new friend, one you want to keep for a lifetime. Certainly, if this friend would need help to lose weight, you'd help. And you'd do so in a positive manner.

Let's say your friend is a woman who wants to have a body that will fit into a size-twelve dress. You wouldn't criticize her and tell her she lacked ability. You'd say, "Go for it! I'm behind you 100 percent."

Get a mental image of yourself in a size-twelve dress, or, if you're a man, in an Armani suit—a strong, intense image you can feel with every cell in your body. Now let your "best friend" help you. Repeat out loud, "I can. I will. I am able to achieve a body that fits a size-twelve dress."

Now comes the work. You must repeat this positive affirmation every day, while holding your vivid mental image. You must repeat it many times over a period of days and weeks until you have created a new, positive subconscious structure that will take the place of the destructive one that told you you were hopeless.

Old habits of negative thinking are firmly embedded

in your mind. It will take time and effort to root them out, then replace them with the can-do attitudes that will change your life.

Be interested in yourself as a friend would. Awaken to your inner needs. Whatever you have to do, do it now and do it well. Then take time to celebrate your own progress. Hear your best friend saying, "You are all the positive things you think you are." Your friend's on the right track.

## What's in Your Way?

To succeed in this most important endeavor of your life, you will need to be wholly committed to learning to think, eat, and live a new way.

Start with what you believe about yourself. Perhaps you think you are star-crossed because something always seems to make you fall short of your diet goal. Maybe you're convinced that you're unworthy of success, that you deserve to fail.

If you think these thoughts, chances are you'll make your prophecies come true. But when you hear, "I can't do that," and your healthy new voice comes right back, "The hell I can't," then your journey is off to a fighting start.

Have you ever had a critical parent or teacher predict that you were bound to fail? Did you get mad and make the opposite come true just to show that person? Try some of this reverse psychology on yourself. If you find your mind divided, with the negative half pulling down the positive half, get mad at your negative self. Become indignant with the half of you that predicts failure, indignant enough to succeed at your new way of living.

It's important to destroy negative thinking for a number of reasons. Sometimes our thoughts can act like a magnet to draw parallel thoughts. When you think unhealthy thoughts, for example, other unhealthy thoughts are attracted to your mind while healthy thoughts are chased away. Take this chain of negative thinking, for instance: "I've failed to lose weight so many times. Now I'm just a big, fat slob, and I don't deserve to be thin. I might as well go ahead and eat." See how one unhealthy thought is attracted by another until there's no chance this person will shed pounds?

Conversely, when you conjure healthy thoughts, unhealthy ones are blocked. For instance: "I'm a worthwhile human being. I deserve to be thin and happy. I'm starting a new eating plan today." What happened? One healthy thought attracted another and another until a thrilling new life opens.

In the following pages, you will find some mind traps you may have fallen into when overeating, or ones that make sticking to a healthy life plan more difficult. These are the specific faulty thinking habits you need to overcome. And they can be beaten by changing to a mental attitude that supports your deepest desire.

*Misinformation*

We overeaters have programmed our minds with so-called facts for so long that we act as if they were true. For example, one struggling dieter reported that every spring she lost control of her eating. The rest of the year she followed a good, nutritious eating plan, but come spring, she regained the weight it had taken her nine months to lose, and then some. Because this person's mind had responded this way before, it responded each spring to the thought that overeating was inevitable. And so it was.

Sometimes you have to walk away from your problem a little to see the answer. Try to step outside the mental image that insists you repeat destructive eating behavior over and over. Take a good look. Do you see any real reason why you must overeat every spring, on weekends, or on certain holidays? Of course there isn't. Remember, you have choices. You are not bound by what you formerly did. This spring (or today), choose a different path.

Misinformation about who we are exists in the labels we stick on ourselves. For example, do you say, "I'm just a fat person without much hope," or, "I'm a thoroughly weak person and I deserve what I get," or, "Since I'm fat, I must have done something terribly wrong"?

Psychologists call this kind of labeling "negative self-hypnosis." It makes us dwell on defeats instead of victories, and we spend a great deal of time convincing ourselves that a thin, healthy body is impossible.

Starting this minute, try the reverse—positive self-hypnosis. Encourage yourself. Don't make sweeping judgments that seem to prove that you are incapable of performing what you want to do. You may have failed in the past, but who knows what you might be capable of in the future?

Today you are better than you were yesterday. And tomorrow you will be better than you are today. You are growing each day. Your capabilities are unlimited.

Look at yourself. You are beginning to think differently. You are responding to many life situations differently. It makes no sense to think you can't accomplish tomorrow what you didn't accomplish yesterday. That bit of misinformation denies the reality of your own growth.

And you *are* growing in your inner self, while your outer body is shrinking to its natural size. When a food temptation comes at you full force, you don't throw up your hands and say, "I have to give in because I used to give in." You stand firm instead: "I'm better every day, so I no longer have to be ruled by appetite."

## Food Fantasies

Recovering alcoholics know that daydreaming too much about the real or imagined pleasures of the bottle increases the likelihood that they will return to drinking. Sober people caution, "Thinking is drinking."

The same is true for overeaters—perhaps even truer. Unlike the alcoholic who must abstain from alcohol, the overeater must eat to live—and three times a day at that. So overeaters must be especially wary of food fantasies. In our case, "Thinking is eating."

"When I started my food plan," one overeater confessed, "I kept a mental list of all the foods I was missing. After a week of daydreaming, I went off my diet, ate my way through the list, and gained twenty-five pounds before I could stop."

Food fantasies, when we dwell on them, ensure that sooner or later we will succumb to these negative temptations. But positive fantasies can be fun and can work to your advantage.

Try closing your eyes and imagining yourself having your clothes altered to a smaller size or buying a youthful new style. Listen to the voices of your friends exclaiming how good you look.

Now focus on the new life you want to live, where excess food is no longer your sole preoccupation. You'll discover this fantasy is the best one you've ever had.

## The Sacrifice Perspective

Focusing on what you're giving up, seeing yourself as making a sacrifice, is a diet-busting attitude. Review your past unsuccessful attempts at losing weight. You will probably find that, often, your thoughts turned to the high-calorie foods you had eliminated from your diet.

Overeaters with long track records of weight-losing diet failures can change the odds in their favor by simply switching their train of thought: *Don't focus on what you are giving up, but on what you are getting.* As one successful weight-loser saw it, "I stopped thinking, 'I can't have that.' Instead, I started thinking, 'I no longer choose to eat that food.'"

For a real eye-opener, take an inventory. When you decide to give yourself a new eating plan for better, more healthful living, what are you really sacrificing? Lonely nights. Guilty days. Clothes that gap and seams that split. Job promotions that go to others. Self-loathing.

Now, what are you gaining? A chance to live closer to yourself and to other people. The energy to work on your real needs. The ability to concentrate without running to food for constant support. A new thin image. Confidence. Inner peace. Getting excess food out of the way of real living is the greatest gift you can give yourself.

## The Pinocchio Complex

In the Italian children's story, the puppet Pinocchio desperately wants to be a real boy, but his habit of lying causes his nose to grow longer with each new lie.

In a similar way, we desperately want to be thin so we can live a more normal life, but because we lie to ourselves about food, our bodies grow bigger with each new lie. Each time we tell ourselves we can have "just one more little bite," we are falling victim to the Pinocchio complex. And like the little puppet, we can't hide our deceptions either.

But we can put an end to the big lie simply by taking responsibility for our eating. We can't kid ourselves that "this piece of cake doesn't matter," or "I'll skip my diet while I'm on vacation, or for Christmas, or for my birthday." With each new deception, we'll grow and grow.

Be honest with yourself—support and help yourself accept the truth. It will get you where you want to go, but first, you have to rid yourself of the Pinocchio complex. Self-deception is difficult to recognize, especially when we lie to make ourselves comfortable with a bad decision. Today, work at self-honesty. It will quickly become part of your life when you get to know yourself and recognize your motives.

*Crutches*

The worst crutch most overeaters lean on is excess food. But often we have other wobbly crutches—flimsy excuses that won't support our desire to lose weight. Do you lean on any of the following excuses:

1. *What will people think if I try a new diet?* This all-purpose crutch can really halt progress. It's fine to be concerned about public opinion, but sometimes you have to swim against the tide to accomplish your goal.

2. *I don't have the time.* Some overeaters console themselves by saying, "It takes too long to do the special shopping and cooking that a diet demands. I should give that extra time to my family, my job, or some worthy cause." Who are you kidding? That extra time will be devoted to overeating. Achievers always have enough time in their day to accomplish what's really important to them.

3. *I'll do it next week when things are better.* Somehow things are never better for procrastinators. There's always a "next week" and the diet (or other needed improvement) never gets started.

4. *Those diets don't ever work for me.* This person is defeated before he or she starts. Such a life contains no enthusiasm. *Don't, can't,* and *won't* are the operative

words, and they carry this dieter nowhere. This is the weakest crutch of all and leaves such people on their knees most of the time.

Using rickety old crutches to prop up a negative personality is a prescription for failure. But crutches can be replaced by sturdy new attitudes: "I *can* succeed no matter what other people think. I *do* have the time, no matter how much time it takes. This week is *always* better than next. And I will find a weight-loss plan that works for me because I will *make* it work.

### Mind Brakes

Our minds have limitless power for change, but sometimes we apply brakes to growth in the form of limiting thought behavior.

There are four ways you apply brakes to your mind, four ways you hamper your own progress.

First, you waste vital energy when you wallow in guilt for past mistakes. It takes an enormous amount of mind power for self-condemnation and self-pity. It puts an absolute brake on your creative thinking processes.

Second, and conversely, you can spend far too much time dwelling on yesterday's successes. An overemphasis on past glories is really an unrecognized fear of the future. Rather than risking an uncertain tomorrow, you're resting on your laurels.

Third, you might use your age as an excuse. When you are young, you are too young; when you are older, you are too old. Age has nothing to do with capability.

Fourth, you don't believe in your potential for personal growth. Many of us project today's problems into the future; then, based on our present knowledge, think tomorrow will be no different. Have faith in your ability to learn. What seems unsolvable today may have a ready answer in the future.

If you think in a limiting way, your mind will have reduced scope and fewer options with which to work. But if you let go of limiting thoughts and behavior, your potential is infinite. So release those negative brakes.

## Great Expectations

Too often the ups and downs that occur when you reform destructive eating patterns get you into a doubting mode. Perhaps fears of failure lurk in the corners of your mind, ready to jump out and mug your confidence. When you think you'll fail or doubt your abilities, you can hardly expect success.

The most important thing for every dieter to practice is an *attitude of expectancy*. Expect the best. Expect that your future is bright and that you will overcome the problem that has you, literally, by the throat.

Of course, shaking off the blues isn't always easy. Self-pity and just plain pessimism can keep expectations low. "How can I eat more healthfully today than I did yesterday?" you ask, doubtfully.

One way is to expect it to be so. Inspirational columnist Doug Hooper says, "In the long run, nobody can stop your succeeding except yourself." Every thought, he goes on, becomes an action according to the strength and desire contained in that thought.

If you expect the best of yourself today, you may surprise yourself with the strength of your ability to act on your desires. If you expect that you will give your best to a better way of eating today, absolutely no one can stop you.

Today is your day for living and choosing. You can learn to use this and every other day of your life creatively and positively. The art of choosing and pursuing your life's goals will release a fantastic energy—coping power. This is the power produced by self-insight and positive thought. It means that you will not be overwhelmed by life problems to the point where you must hold yourself together with one food binge after another. You will be able to cope with events as they come along. You will expect the best, and when you do, wonderful things will begin to happen.

*Happiness*

According to psychologist Erich Fromm, happiness is an *achievement* brought about by inner productiveness. People succeed at being happy, he says, by building a liking for themselves, and they like themselves in direct proportion to how close they get to what they want. Fromm then sums it up by adding, "Happiness is proof of success in the art of living."

The following suggestions may help you to unlearn self-defeating behavior:

1. *Stop playing assumed roles.* If you're acting out the "jolly fat person" role, stop and instead be *you.* You can't people-please your way to happiness.

2. *Take risks.* If you want to change, don't let anxiety stop you. Change sometimes involves fear but little actual personal danger. And what if you fail? You can always try again.

3. *Don't blame others.* Stop saying, "My mother made me fat," or "My boss makes me feel bad." Replace blaming others with self-responsibility.

4. *Assert yourself.* You're a grown-up. Don't ask others how you should lead your life. Decide for yourself.

5. *Don't analyze.* Give why a rest. Several times each day, allow your brain to rest.

6. *Don't look to others for validation of your self-worth.* People resent it, and you won't believe what they say anyhow. Ironically, the less you ask for approval, the more you'll receive it.

7. *Associate with positive people.* They will expect you to be happy, too, and their influence will affect you.

It is so much easier to feel satisfaction as you moderate your eating and restructure your life. No matter what your other achievements, it was awfully hard to admire yourself when you were overeating.

Feeling a glow of happiness is a wonderful change in your life and you appreciate it, but how can you keep that glow alive? The answer is clear: keep on keeping on. Continued happiness is based on a sense of purpose and on striving toward that purpose. "Ah, but a man's reach should exceed his grasp, or what's a heaven for?" wrote poet Robert Browning.

Often, we don't think beyond our reach. We downgrade our abilities to achieve; sometimes we even adopt a "what the hell" stance and give up. But surrender is not for someone who seeks a happy life.

Strive. Push yourself. Never let yourself give up on you. Every day is another potentially happy day that you can make happen—another new day of food control for health. Such days are learning days, achieving days, beautiful in-control, thin days. Happy days.

*Peace*

Why do you want to lose weight? You can think of a dozen obvious reasons, and we've gone over quite a few of them. But there's another reason which isn't so obvious: *peace.* Some call it contentment, consciousness, or even God.

Despite all the stuffing of food, overweight people still suffer an emptiness, a strange blank spot that food never fills. If you dig deep for the priceless treasure of a slender, healthy body, you will discover another precious prize: inner peace and contentment. You will simply no longer be fighting yourself.

When you are drowning in repeated acts of overeating, you block wonderful positive experiences. They may even be happening to you, but you can't feel them. You are only capable of feeling pain, suffering, disgust, and tension. You can't get to your creative inner self until you remove the excess food. And when you do, you'll meet your positive, joyful inner self—your truth, love, joy, and beauty.

Today, try to function from the inside out. When you feel good, try to become as one with the feeling. Let go of the inhibiting blocks of fear, doubt, reservation, and self-criticism.

Live today as if today were the most important day in your life. Treat your body with respect—as if how you eat today is the most important thing in your life. You have an obligation to yourself, an obligation to live life to the fullest. Don't accept less than your best. Follow your healthful plan of eating, and stretch your inner self in some new direction. Do so and make a tremendous discovery: the treasure of a life at peace with yourself.

*Freedom*

In order to free yourself from the prison built by compulsive eating, you must first know what true freedom is. *Freedom is obedience to our inner law,* the one that seeks healthy expression through us. We abuse the law of nature when we are overweight and unhealthy, and conflict results, both physically and emotionally.

Freedom must seem desirable before it is possible. Think of *freedom* as another word for *security, stability, progress,* and *creativity.* Are these the attributes of food slaves? Of course not.

True freedom consists in knowing ourselves—our thoughts, motives, desires, and behavior. Without freedom there can be no creation, no self-mastery. And most of all, without freedom there can be no personal happiness because there is no room for change. All growth is stifled.

Freedom is discovering your own way—the wonderful way to live free from the overwhelming desire to eat compulsively. You are beginning to experience freedom as you build, day by day, a master plan of living in harmony with self and others.

*Acceptance*

Many of us who share an eating problem tend to worry about things we can do nothing about—and then we make our situation worse by eating because of them. Here's a good lesson in accepting what you can't change: *If life hands you lemons, make lemonade!* In other words, learn to make the best of what you have.

That doesn't mean you can't create or innovate—just the opposite. Spend less time flailing against the inevitable, and you'll have more time for what you can do something about—or better yet, what you want to do.

Acceptance brings opportunities and solutions; without it you can convince yourself that your future is out of your control and your life is empty. You can easily become too serious about living. Don't forget to enjoy yourself and have fun! It's important to be determined and serious in your weight loss, but not "deadly" serious. Even if we simply *act as if* we're happy, we will be.

Losing weight and revealing the new person beneath that excess flesh is a joyful experience. When your clothes begin to droop, when your rings start to fall off, *that's fun.* And what's more joyous than walking into a department store and buying the latest style in a smaller size?

But that's only the beginning of the real fun. No longer will tender, sensitive feelings block out the joy of life, the sheer delight of living in a body that is really alive.

Accept this day with its ups and its downs, and let the pleasure in it spill into every minute. You're free from feelings of heaviness, from the need to be perfect, from the weight of the world. Your sense of well-being and ease with yourself will be apparent to everyone you meet.

*Enthusiasm*

Are you eagerly anticipating today? If you can put some honest enthusiasm into your life, it will be far more exciting.

One of the best ways to become vibrant and alive is to get rid of "fat thinking." The main component of fat thinking is the false belief that excess food is necessary. Like an alcoholic who can't imagine having fun at a party without liquor, compulsive eaters can't imagine a day without sweets to soothe their way.

Another component of fat thinking is playing a role to please others. Sometimes, we are the "jolly" fat man or woman. Sometimes we settle for any kind of relationship we can get. Sometimes we become foils for other people's emotional problems.

As you lose extra pounds, you'll find people's attitudes toward you change. It takes time for your own mental image to catch up to your new physical self, but soon you won't find it necessary to play the role of jolly clown or fawning foil. Now you can be your real self.

With fat thinking gone, real enthusiasm will enter your daily life. You will greet each day with exuberance and confidence. Many of us have always had the capacity to be enthusiastic, exciting people, but we allowed food problems to desensitize us to the positive things in our world. No more. As one happy young weight-loser put it, "I never thought being alive could be so much fun." Now that's enthusiasm!

## Pass It On

Sane eating to lose weight or to maintain your target weight is the most important thing in your life. If you have grown new, healthy attitudes, you'll feel this and more.

You are also growing in the willingness to build a positive eating program. Old habits of blaming other people or citing other problems as an excuse to overeat are gone. You feel beautiful, intelligent, and confident. You have serenity of mind and your emotions are balanced, and that makes living a joy. Nothing can happen today that you can't handle. Today you are good for you. But you can make a good day even better.

Most of us dealing with an out-of-control appetite get bogged down with the problems of dieting and living. What's the best way to get off this treadmill? Change your luck. Get out of your problem and spread a little happiness. It's contagious and you'll find others are apt to catch it. What has spreading happiness got to do with losing weight? Just this: It's the best way to make yourself happy, and you won't be as likely to need food.

Do something kind and unexpected today. Give someone your time, your friendship, your ideas. Look for opportunities to do something that will make another person feel good. You could make someone's whole day by simply saying, "You're terrific!" or by doing one of the following:

- Talk of health, happiness, and opportunity to everyone, and most of all to yourself.
- Show your friends there is something in them you really love.
- Think only the best, work for the best, and expect the best for yourself and others.

- Be enthusiastic about your new lifestyle and believe in your ultimate success.
- Give so much time to your inner growth that you won't have time to criticize others or yourself.
- Be truly cheerful.
- Be too full of growing for worry about the future, too forgiving to be angry, too courageous to be fearful, and too happy to permit defeat.

Sometimes you can give happiness and never say a word. A hug, a smile, a friendly pat on the back may be all that's needed to spread happiness—happiness that will turn around and come back to you.

There is a bonus for your good deeds. While you are searching for ways to give yourself away, you can't possibly take the time to overeat or worry that you have an eating problem.

You know enough about yourself to understand that you want to know more. Whatever is ahead, you have the strength to accomplish it—and the health to carry it out.

You've begun to change your thinking. Now you're ready for a quality life.

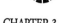

# CHAPTER 3

## Positive Feeling

### Changing Your Self-Concept

*F*eelings are simply your thoughts turned into emo-tions. They are the end product of your opinions and attitudes. Once you have learned the principles of pos-itive thinking, it's time to think of your mind in another way, as the feeding ground for your feelings.

If your mind harbors bitter, sarcastic, unpleasant thoughts, your affirmative feelings will be painfully sti-fled, and crippling negative feelings will emerge. But if your thinking is positive, generous, and empowering, so is your feeling heart. Do you see how uncomplicated the positive life can be? It's outwardly simple, but inwardly rich and fun.

If you make such positive simplicity your thinking/ feeling goal, you will have committed yourself to an easier life, one in which you spend less life-time on damage control and more life-time on creating and *being*. For people with eating problems, that extra time is enormously important. We've got bodies to rebuild and thin new lives to forge.

As you read the following pages and begin to learn how your feelings can help you win, commit to moni-toring yourself each day with a feelings checklist. You probably do this already each morning in front of the mirror. But from now on, keep track of the negative and positive emotions you feel as you face yourself. Don't be critical, just honest, because this knowledge will give you power to change. Take a good look. Are you having obsessive feelings about what you're going to eat next? Are you dredging up old hurts, planning revenge, belittling yourself, or buying into other negative feelings?

Now, take another look at the reflection looking back at you. Peer beyond the surface image to get a glimpse of the person you long to be. You'll see positive attributes there, your best qualities, and most important, you'll discover absolute answers to the destructive feelings that have you missing the grand opportunities of your life.

And these positive qualities, which you have possessed all along, are natural tools that can help you. Here are some ways in which you can make these tools work for you:

- First, *use your feelings of love* to look at yourself and your own situation with affection. Hate only reinforces what you see wrong with yourself, and you've focused too long on your overeating and weight gain already.

- *Use your feelings of honesty* to stop hiding from your weight. Lying to yourself is a self-defeating behavior; accepting the truth means you no longer have to overeat to cover up the lie. You know what you weigh, and it's hurting you to hide it.

- *Use your feelings of sensitivity* to be kind to yourself today. Self-hate is the worst diet companion you can have. You wouldn't wish it on your worst enemy.

- *Use your feelings of purpose* to help you move along the road toward your weight goal. People who possess purpose and goals in their lives are working toward solving their problem, and that's the kind of person you want to be.

- Finally, *use your spiritual feelings,* which tell you that you are not alone. You have a Higher Power, or a family and friends, or a group of other overeaters who will help you focus on your affirmative feeling assets.

After recognizing your powerful positive tools, name what feelings you want to make important in your life. Negative or positive? What feelings will help you survive emotionally and make you a healthy winner? It's not much of a contest. Negative feelings will only keep you in the same old binge/diet mode. They will keep you running away from the authentic, thin person you really are.

You already know that your real struggle doesn't take place as you walk past your favorite bakery. Your real struggle occurs in your thoughts and feelings about yourself and the world around you. What happens to you doesn't really count; what counts is what you think and feel about what happens to you. And then whether you eat over it—or not!

A healthy, slender, happy you won't appear magically as the result of iron willpower. Your new body will be the result of your growing into the self-honest, self-loving, self-actualizing person you want to be.

In this chapter, you will learn to build a network of affirming new feelings that will help you control your eating instead of being controlled by it. Through these self-searching and self-watching techniques, you'll find an answer to the haunting question: How do I shed fat and live thin for the rest of my life?

You will learn nothing less than how to take good care of yourself.

## Your Right to Happiness

You have decided where you want to go, and you're learning how to get there. Now you need another resource to take you all the way to being thin and happy: a powerful new ally—*your own affirmative feelings about yourself.*

This positive ally reminds you to believe in your *absolute right* to happiness, fulfilled dreams, and a joy-filled, quality life. Six key tools that are already a part of your positive, creative mind, which can help you claim those rights.

1. *Affection.* You are entitled to love, especially from yourself. Be good to yourself. Keep a journal and mark down the moment you wake up to the fact that *you matter.*

2. *Respect.* It's funny when Rodney Dangerfield says, "I don't get no respect," but it's no joke when this is your sad theme. Stop downgrading your abilities. Start recognizing yourself as a worthy human being.

3. *Skills.* Everyone has special talents, including you. Do your best to develop them. Using your skills will energize your mind, body, and soul.

4. *Knowledge.* You need to learn about nutrition and exercise to live the thin life. Give yourself the opportunity to acquire this knowledge.

5. *Power.* You may have the ability to make powerful business decisions. You may run a community, a club, or a home. But if you can't manage your food problem, you're not using the power you have for your own benefit. Take control of your own life.

6. *Self-realization.* Wanting and dreaming of a new body is not enough. The greatest gift you can give yourself is to realize your dreams. This is how you will find real meaning and satisfaction in life.

Review these six innate tools often. They add up to the ultimate prize you can bestow on yourself—self-esteem.

*Fall in Love—with Yourself*

Over the years, self-love has been given bad press. An early example is the Greek account of Narcissus, who was punished for falling in love with his own reflection. Today's social and religious teachings continue the prohibition. We are supposed to lavish love on others, but be sparing with love for ourselves. Too often, overeaters happily comply. After all, it's easy to withhold love for ourselves when we're overweight, unhappy, unhealthy, and generally feel worthless.

We need to stop hating ourselves for the shape of our bodies and to begin changing our lives (and ultimately our shapes). The first step is to overcome all the old negative feelings, so that we can love ourselves for our very real accomplishments and for the wonderful people we are—regardless of our weight.

Don't be afraid of self-love. It's not just all right; it's an absolute necessity to achieving your target weight. For the dieter, self-love is added energy. Self-love gives us a reason to seek health.

It's one thing to talk about falling in love with ourselves. But how can we really follow through with it? We often feel so unlovable. After all, aren't we the physical opposite of what lovable is supposed to be?

The idea of falling in love with yourself might even sound silly—if it weren't so important. It's urgent because *everything* in your life evolves from the way you see yourself. Unless you care, weight loss or weight maintenance and inner growth won't happen. It is also essential to love yourself before you can truly love another human being. *Real love is love between equals.*

Learning to love yourself is a process. We take small steps toward it rather than plunging in head first. Begin by trying to be patient about your rate of weight loss. There is nothing more individual than your body's response to calories. Next, treat yourself with the same kindness you show other people. Give yourself the attention you need. Of course, you'll continue to care about family and friends, but don't ignore yourself in the process. And stop getting mad at yourself for every minor misstep you might make.

Finally, act with sincerity and integrity. If you promised to change your life and have started to do so, you're building a mighty fortress of self-trust.

These vital elements express your personal love. When you act on them, you will strengthen your ability to succeed.

### Gold at the End of the Rainbow

You have the power to change your world by redirecting your feelings. If you dislike yourself because of your weight problem or your eating behavior, the power of your negative feelings can give you a bitter outlook on life. But when you develop a favorable opinion of yourself, you see gold at the end of the rainbow. Maintaining this positive outlook will bring many rewards. One pay-off is lost pounds. You'll also enjoy your own company more. And the more you like your own company, the less vulnerable you'll be to outside criticism.

*You are good.* Once you accept this premise, you'll be on your way. Of course, we all have faults, things we must work on. But you're not the worthless slob you may have been telling yourself you are.

Have you realistically assessed your abilities and your potential? You already know that you have the ability to lose extra pounds and to live in a healthy, happy body. You know you can reach your goals by taking one step at a time, one day at a time, even though at times it seems as though they exceed your reach and demand your best. Remember that your best is good enough.

In former days we felt like failures, like meaningless blobs of flesh. We were but a short step from feeling to feeding. But now that we feel we are *good,* we have the ability to succeed at life's tasks. Now we can move forward and do more for ourselves by eating less. Each success we enjoy is another step toward the gold at the end of the rainbow—a healthy, happy life.

*Through the Looking Glass*

"Self-actualization" is a term used by the human potential movement to describe the continuing struggle to become what you *know* you are. Actualizing yourself is like declaring your own independence—proclaiming your own life, liberty, and pursuit of happiness. It is an attempt to find the *whole* you. Like the fictional Alice, you can stand before a looking glass and discover a wonderland in the reflection.

For overeaters, self-actualization is visualizing yourself the way you can be. Somehow, when we look at ourselves, the extra pounds cover more than just our real shape. They obliterate our human potential; they hide our abilities and skills. We must escape from underneath our flesh before we can begin to fully realize who we can be.

This visualization process is not an exercise in seeking perfection. It is the way we discover our own internal truths. It is a way of achieving daily fulfillment and self-knowledge.

The process of self-realization is not a speedy one. It will take you longer than a day, perhaps more than a month, but it will be worth every hour it takes. The day will come when you will have forged a new power in the center of your self, and that power will help you reshape your whole life.

The longer we search for self-knowledge, the more natural this new way of living seems and the more we realize that our old overeating lives were unnatural, physically and mentally. At first we wondered how we could possibly live without our food crutch. But as we learn more and more about our own capabilities, we are discovering that we can rely on ourselves. Isn't this the wonderland we've been wanting?

## You Are Your Own Master

All people, thin or fat, have one desire in common—the desire to control their own lives. It is a comfort to know that living need not be a matter of fate or luck, that we as individuals can have a deciding hand in it.

You gain the ability to take control when your mind and heart believe that what you desire can become real. This principle works for health, self-fulfillment, success, freedom from anxiety, and building better relationships. What you can do with your mind in building a thinner, healthier image of yourself, you can also do for many other areas of your life.

The first step in taking control of your life is to get acquainted with your own thoughts and feelings. You can do this by meditating or by spending simple, quiet times with yourself. These are your listening times. And the more you tune in, the more you come to believe in the strength of your own mind.

Give yourself some time each day to let your positive mind power and the positive feelings it generates work for you and for whatever problem you want to tackle. Trust this power, and it will become increasingly effective.

Once you've learned to harness this creative mind power, you can use it to take control of your body and your weight. Eastern philosophies and religions call this "self-mastery": through the use of diet, meditation, and ritual, control is gained over body, mind, and emotions. You can practice using your self-mastery skills by doing exercises such as the following:

Repeat the phrase "I am the master of my body." Sit in a quiet place and feel that you are the master of your body. Continue to say the phrase to yourself over and over again.

Then without allowing intrusive thoughts, feel and visualize that you are the master of your body. Really know that you are the superior of your physical self, all the while visualizing and feeling exactly what you eventually want to be like. This is important because what you create now, you create in your future.

Think of that! *What you visualize now is your future.* Every little bit of positive affirmation you awaken today adds up to a more promising future. Don't just try to master your body. Repeat the previous exercise with your mind and emotions as well. Repeat over and over, "I am the master of my body, my mind, and my emotions."

If you have always told yourself, "I'm fat, and there's nothing much I can do about it," reexamine that assumption. It is untrue. You can do something about it. You are the master of your body, your mind, and your emotions.

### A Valuable Value System

Hand in hand with coming to love yourself is coming to value yourself—discovering your self-worth. The late psychologist Virginia Satir, author of *Conjoint Family Therapy,* developed a list of personality styles that tells us a great deal about how different types of people view themselves in terms of self-esteem. Can you identify with any of the styles?

1. The *placater* says, "I'm worthless, you're worthy." This is a feeling we overweight people often find ourselves expressing. We assume that if other people are thin, they automatically are worthier than us, since fat is "bad."

2. The *blamer* says, "I'm worthy, you're worthless." This person is an attacker, always accusing others of being at fault. He or she is a finger-pointer. The blamer says, "My mother made me fat," even after being responsible for his or her own eating for twenty years.

3. The *calculator* says, "I'm not worthy, but you're not worthy either." This person believes that all people should sacrifice themselves to a cause or circumstance.

4. The *distracter* says, "Nothing is worth anything." Distracters never share themselves because, basically, they feel unworthy. When distracters are fat they will often say, "What's the use?"

5. The *actualizer,* conversely, has a value system that's useful. The actualizer says, "Everything has worth." Most of us overweight people aren't there yet, but we're working toward becoming actualizers. We share feelings and support each other. We take ourselves and others seriously. We are honest. We take risks because that is the way we grow.

When you develop a sense of self-worth, you will start thinking of yourself as beautiful. Right now, you may define beauty as perfect features coupled with a perfect body, but you'll soon realize that beauty is more than this. All of us have a great deal of beauty in our lives, and we easily can have more.

Good adjustment is beauty; it is anything that has unity. Your healthful way of eating is a good adjustment. And that is beautiful.

Faith is beauty. And you have an instinctive faith in your future, which springs from within.

And finally, truth is beauty. Whether you like it or not, you come face to face with truth whenever you step on your scale. Eventually, even weighing your body will be a beautiful experience.

*First Things First*

Everyone knows that the human body has a basic need for air, food, and water. But once we've taken care of these basics, we need to go one step further and sustain our emotional selves.

For overweight people, meeting emotional needs often means increasing self-esteem. The key to self-esteem is to bring your feelings about yourself into line with the lifestyle you want. The closer you get to your ideal self, the higher your self-esteem rises. In other words, the more you live your life as you feel you should, the more you like yourself.

Why not try acting as if you are the person you want to be? Eat like a person who cares about weight and nutrition. Act like a person who lives an optimistic and winning life. Gradually, as you move in a more positive direction, your self-esteem will rise. And this heightened self-esteem will pave the way to inner peace.

The way to inner peace has been defined as right thought, right feeling, and right action. These are the requisites for harmony, which is the absence of conflict. To have peace of mind, we must seek a beautiful relationship with our inner selves. All distortions, restlessness, and incoherence must be replaced by the positive, creative mind.

No one else can give us the sense of unity and cohesion that stills conflict. We must give it to ourselves each day by creating a constructive environment in which to live.

*Remove Your Blinders*

If there's one thing on which the saints and great teachers of the ages agree, it's on the concept that human beings should seek self-knowledge. Trying to live in a complex world without this essential information is like living with blinders on—you don't know where you are, can't see where you are going, and place yourself in danger with every step.

But now you are growing daily in self-knowledge, and you have come to a state of peace within yourself. Enough, perhaps, to be honest. Give yourself permission to look deep inside. Help yourself to focus by asking these three questions:

1. *What kind of person am I?* Don't just think of your physical self, but your personality as well. If you had to describe yourself in one phrase, what positive statement could you make to sell yourself to the world? Write down that statement.

2. *What are my good points?* Make a list of six of your positive personality traits. Now take a good look at your list—those traits are something to be proud of.

3. *What positive things do other people say about me?* Write down all the positive things you have been told, overheard, or sensed that indicate the way others react positively to you.

Now look at your list. Aren't you impressed? All of those people could not have been wrong—you are a good person.

This exercise gives us some tools we need to communicate positively with ourselves. Positive self-communication helps us triumph over negative feelings and, ultimately, over our weight problem. It can also mean finding hidden talents that lie unnoticed under all the negativity.

Self-communication is a form of prayer with yourself. When your communications are positive, the result is positive feeling, and that is another word for *faith*. And when you have faith, anything is possible.

Remove the blinders that have kept you in the dark for so long. In the light you can get to know your true self—not the fearful you, stumbling in perpetual night, but the confident, self-assured you.

Begin by throwing away the assumption that nothing can be done about your weight problem. That is a false belief you have been nurturing in the blackness of self-deception. You have an innate ability to change your life, to become the slim person who is your inner ideal.

In a manner similar to the previous exercise, take an inventory of the positive and powerful things you do every day. This positive inventory will alter any lingering feeling that you are somehow a sad victim of fate. And this self-knowledge will strengthen you in the fight against overeating.

As you learn to deal positively with the anxieties of your everyday life, you are learning more about yourself. You are becoming more aware of and are learning to deal with the feelings that you formerly masked with too much food. The inevitable result is that you will have an ever-increasing ability to control your appetite.

Remember, no one changes a lifelong way of reacting overnight. Growth will be gradual, but it *will* happen. Each time you conquer a negative feeling that once would have driven you to the refrigerator, you are stronger for the next confrontation.

You are stronger each time you win a small battle against self-hate, hopelessness, and guilt. The day will come when you are so strong; self-hate will have been rooted out.

*The Magic in Self-Acceptance*

Each time you accept yourself, even when you discover things you'd rather not face, you grow, and you become more accepting the next time. Self-knowledge helps you live with your mistakes, learn from them, and then let go of them.

Let go. Let it be. Let it happen. In this case, the word *let* is not a passive word. It implies an active and trusting acceptance of life. It means allowing your own affection to come to the fore instead of being manipulated by a negative will. It means permitting your own natural beauty to touch you instead of manufacturing a dark outcome you think you deserve.

Let the good life happen to you. Try to get in touch with the person you really are—your inner love and, yes, your beauty. As you practice new and healthy ways of eating, believe that what is happening inside you is as important as what is happening outside you.

In your head, you carry around an image of the kind of person you want to be. So when your behavior, especially your eating behavior, doesn't measure up to your idea, you become depressed, disappointed, and cease to trust yourself. But this is your past; the future will be different.

By acting as if you are already the person you want to be, a day will come when you'll look in the mirror and say, "I know you." Personal joy will come from knowing that from the depths of once-uncontrollable overeating, you have risen to such self-knowledge and self-control. You are all the good things you feel you are. It's your thinking and feeling that must change more than your being.

The days ahead won't always be easy, yet you will be surprised when you pick yourself right up and begin again after a stumble. You will find friends who give you help and love. When you are afraid, you will find courage. When you feel guilty, you will find forgiveness. When you feel self-pity, you will find perseverance.

## When the Going Gets Tough

It's easy to have faith in yourself and feel self-worth when you're winning. It's not so easy on days when you've overeaten, when you feel lethargic and beaten, and when the road ahead seems too hard and too long.

These are the times when you will need to fan the fires of faith even harder. Remember that you can change your life a little at a time, and momentary setbacks will only give you more strength for the future.

The old saying "Where there's life, there's hope" conveys a great truth for overweight people. Nobody hangs on to that hope more than we do. But before we can *really* believe it, we have to put ourselves in the right frame of mind by improving our concept of ourselves.

Strange as it sounds, overweight people who lose their excess weight often still think of themselves as fat. Usually the problem begins when they are within a few pounds of their target weight. At that time, many people start having doubts. They fear their ability to maintain their new weight, or they feel they can't cope with their improved physical image. Most of all, they feel that living the disciplined life of a thin person will be too tough.

But such doubts can be overcome. One successful weight-loser, who has kept one hundred pounds off for twenty years, shares the strategy he used to keep his weight-loss plan on track: first, he identified all his bad eating habits and then set about to remove them one by one. Twice a day he found a quiet place and systematically relaxed every muscle in his body. During this state of calm, he felt his subconscious become extremely susceptible to suggestion.

"I didn't try to empty my mind," he says. "Instead, I imagined my mind was a telescope and focused it smaller and smaller until I was seeing only one mental image. Then I began to make mental pictures of myself reaching for celery and other low-calorie foods, instead of candy. I even watched myself *enjoy* celery."

Finally, to help him keep the weight off, he set about to rid himself of his self-image of a fat man. Like many overweight people, he envisioned himself as fat. With this mental picture, he was programmed to act like a fat person, which meant eating like one too.

Each day, he worked at reprogramming his mind, imagining himself looking thinner and wearing smaller clothing. By the time he lost all of his excess weight, he looked thin not only in the mirror, but in his mind as well.

As you approach your target weight, you need to work on your new thin image. You've been feeling fat for a long time. Now it's time to feel thin. Compare photos shot before you started losing weight with ones taken recently. Place them side by side. See the difference? Next, check your tape-measure records. You can't argue with those figures.

Finally, if you still have a problem thinking and feeling thin, take positive action. Ask your doctor or weight group to set up a meeting with others having a similar image crisis. You'll find, firsthand, how others are overcoming this mental block. And best of all, you'll come to understand that your feelings are all too normal.

**What You Think Is How You Feel**

Depressed people almost always describe themselves in negative terms. They can't even escape in their dreams, and often dream that they are frustrated, humiliated, rejected, deprived, or punished. What over-weight child hasn't dreamed of being ridiculed by class-mates? What adult overweight person hasn't dreamed of being rejected because of size? How often have you told yourself: "I am dumb, I am lazy, I am fat, I can't finish anything"?

Instead of reinforcing these untrue beliefs, set up an internal dialogue with yourself to combat these views. For example, when you say, "I am dumb," ask yourself how you have managed to hold down a responsible job for so many years. When you say, "I am fat," answer with the positive acts you are taking to lose weight and be healthy. Continue with this internal dialogue until you have reached realistic conclusions you can believe and feel. When you *think* positively about yourself, you'll *feel* positively about yourself.

It takes a concentrated effort to change habits, responses, and beliefs. One simple way to begin is to change the language you use about yourself in your internal dialogue and with others. For instance, many dieters overuse loaded terms such as *sin, failure,* and *bad* in describing unsuccessful dieting efforts—and them-selves. In effect, the use of such language leaves them with a sense of moral stigma—an unnecessary burden for people already overburdened with society-induced guilt.

Switch to success words in your dialogues. Begin referring to yourself as *confident, courageous, under-standing, accepting, goal-oriented, creative, loving, thor-ough, hard-working, attractive, honest, strong, willing, open-minded, persistent, determined,* and *faithful.* Not only will you improve your vocabulary, you'll also be taking a step toward thinking—and thus feeling—more positive about yourself.

*Nobody's Perfect*

At one time or another you've excused a friend's mistake with the comforting words, "Don't worry. Nobody's perfect," and you really meant it. It's too harsh to shower blame on someone who is already down. You understand this, yet how often have you said this to yourself and really meant it?

Most of us suffer from anxiety and guilt over imagined mistakes or over our own exaggerated standards. We forget that making mistakes is only part of being human. People with food problems tend to be perfectionists in the rest of their lives. In a way, we're saying, "Don't look at our bodies, look at what we do so well." But perfectionism is an intolerable burden. It requires us to be unkind, impatient, and intolerant with ourselves.

What's the answer? Simply this: Try having the *courage to be imperfect*. If you don't demand perfection from yourself, your life will immediately become more manageable. The next time you don't meet the standards you've set, treat yourself as you'd treat a friend. Tell yourself softly, "Don't worry. Nobody's perfect." And really mean it.

A perfectionist attitude toward losing weight sets you up for failure. The perfectionist says, "One slip and it's all over." This all-or-nothing attitude gives you permission to fail because it's easier than coping with mistakes.

Challenge perfectionism. Instead of going on an eating binge after every little dietary mistake, be realistic. Allow yourself to make mistakes, and learn from them. If your eating plan is a good one, get a second opinion about why you are having difficulty sticking to it. Call a fellow dieter or even your doctor. You will learn that other dieters have problems equal to yours. We have to learn to be persistent, not perfect. And we do better when we get out of our own way.

If you consistently fall short of your goals, don't judge yourself to be a failure. Perhaps your goals are unrealistic. For example, if you tell yourself, "I must lose one pound a day," the first day you don't lose the allotted pound, your self-esteem takes a nosedive. Worse yet, out of anger or spite you may overeat and regain the prior week's loss.

You deserve your own good will, and from that, you can grow in true self-love and self-esteem. So take it easy. Even treat yourself a little. When you find yourself caught up in the everyday demands of a "perfectionist" life, give your mind a break. Use your imagination to conjure a peaceful scene where you have no demands and no worries, and escape to that place for a few minutes. When you return, you'll be free of undue anxiety and perfectionistic attitudes. You'll be better able to cope with your day, whatever it brings.

Anxiety caused by perfectionism delivers a double whammy to dieters. It not only keeps your performance level low, but it sabotages your ideal plan of living and eating. And how many of us have held down anxiety with a heavy layer of extra food?

Take it easy. Find a quiet, secluded place of your own and take a little vacation. You deserve one.

### You Are Not a Weight

Those of us fighting a lifelong battle against the desire for more food than our body needs have a problem of personal identity. "I can remember what I weighed on almost every day of my adult life," confessed one overeater. "I can't remember some significant things I did, but I can tell you, to the pound, what I weighed."

Know this: You are not a weight. Like everyone, you are a paradoxical mix of all human attributes and weaknesses. You are loving and hateful, generous and greedy, courageous and fearful, energetic and lazy—but you are *not* just a weight.

You are also more than a body. You are a human being with feelings. The answer to every emotion is not more eating—it is allowing yourself to experience your feelings. The answer to anger is to feel angry. Don't eat. The answer to sadness is to feel sad. Don't eat. The answer to disappointment is to feel new resolve. Begin again, and don't eat.

Becoming aware of the ways you have used food in your life will show you how to change your habits. For instance, you may have used extra food to avoid dealing with your feelings—allowing walls of cookies to separate your feelings from your ability to act positively on those feelings.

Recognizing this, you can take one bold step forward and try to modify your eating habits today. The next time you're experiencing intense feelings, you can consciously decide to avoid numbing them with food and instead go for a walk or call a friend to give yourself time to work through the feelings.

Have you decided that you prefer a good life? Have you become more open to change? Now you know that you're more than a weight or a body; you are a creative mind. You have an arsenal of solutions to your living problems.

Soon a thinner, more healthful body will emerge from behind our fat cover-ups. But first we must honestly face these outer images—those that objectify or limit us.

What is your ideal image? Look into the mirror of your mind and scan that image. Erase the extra flesh around your lower jaw, upper arms, abdomen, and thighs. Do you have this new image firmly in mind? Hold it there.

Remember that today is another day you can give yourself to become that slender image you really are. Keep constantly in your thoughts the physical image of how great you really look. You already have this ideal size and shape, if you will just uncover it. You already are what you want to be, but you must strip away the outer fat that hides you.

*Self-Worth Is Waiting for You*

So often, we tell ourselves, "When I'm thin I'll go swimming" or, "When I look fabulous, I'll buy new clothes." We make the simple pleasures and even necessities of life dependent on how much we weigh, but we need to take pride in ourselves today, just as we are.

Fight the idea that you must lose all your excess weight *before* you feel self-worth. Having feelings of pride and self-worth are important for you right now. On your way to a more desirable and healthful weight, there's no reason to postpone living the way you want to live, wearing what you want to wear, and doing what you want to do. Your weight-loss goal is worth working and waiting for. Only you or someone who's been through it can possibly appreciate what a struggle it is to become thin. But your struggle leaves more than a new figure in its wake. It teaches you to like yourself, to take good care of yourself, and, above all, to enjoy your life. And this feeling of self-worth is *not* something to wait for. You deserve to feel it now.

Let go of any limiting feelings about yourself, as you are today. You needn't hide extra pounds under extra clothes. You know (whether anyone else knows or not) that one day at a time you are working toward your new image, inside and outside. You believe in your ultimate success. You are determined and enthusiastic.

Feel free to let this enthusiasm spill over into the outside world, and be ready for positive feedback from your friends and family. We overweight people are conditioned to making excuses in the wake of negative feedback. We don't always know how to respond when what comes back to us is good. We tend to minimize our accomplishments and positive attributes.

Many of us have such scant self-regard that we can turn a genuine compliment into a personal put-down. Sometimes we program ourselves to reject the honest admiration of others. We feel we can't do anything right. This negative feeling is not even rational.

You do many things well. You deserve every compliment you get. If you wish to become a more gracious receiver, try practicing some self-compliments. If you perform a task well, tell yourself so. If your hair, outfit, or face looks particularly attractive today, give yourself a compliment.

What's the right way to respond to a compliment? Say *thank you*. That's all.

*Replacing Labels*

Some people are given labels early in life that, later on, are hard to change. For example, if you develop a reputation as the family spendthrift when you're young, it doesn't matter how you may mature into fiscal responsibility; some people will always assign the "family wastrel" role to you.

Sometimes you assign your own labels. For example, Jane was the typical jolly fat wife. "I'm shade in the summer," she laughed, "and heat in the winter." From the act she put on even in front of her fellow weight-group members, it was hard to guess that Jane was really hurting. "I had to make a public joke about my weight," she recalled later, "before someone else did. I was just protecting myself with humor."

Overweight people are often afflicted with the "good sport syndrome." We participate in our own humiliation because we think it's inappropriate not to do so. While a sense of humor, especially about oneself, is important, it should be *humor with dignity.* The result? You will gain self-esteem, you will feel less ill at ease, and you will feel more self-assured.

It's bad enough when others label us and try to keep us confined to our labels long after we've outgrown them, but it's even worse when we do that to ourselves. Sometimes we hang on to old labels because they are comfortable or because we get a sympathetic reaction from others. We say, "Oh, I'm really not very thrifty," or "I'm just Mr. Five-by-Five." Cruel old labels can have us in a stranglehold. However, by repeating our good changes and good experiences, we can reidentify ourselves.

You need to build your self-assurance every day by affirming that a change has taken place. One way to affirm change is through repetition. If you are *repeatedly* eating healthfully and not playing your old "fat role," then you can use this repetition to develop a new self-image.

Be aware that your behavior has changed, and don't deny positive experiences. Suppose you went clothes shopping twice and both times returned with an outfit one size smaller. These are positive experiences. Allow them to reinforce your changing body image.

Stop limiting yourself to old roles. Encourage yourself in new, more positive ones. Believe only what you want to live: no more jolly, fat labels, no more jokes at your own expense.

## Lessons from the Outside World

You can get to know yourself better by holding up a mirror to your own behavior. But it also helps to look at other people's behavior. Feedback from these two sources will give you the insight you need to revolutionize your own patterns of overeating.

You don't have to be a psychologist to study behavior. The more insight into behavior you gain, the more warning signals you pick up. For example, identifying which foods you tend to binge on is an insight that can lead to a change in behavior. Then the next time you are tempted by your binge foods, you can send a "stop" signal from your mind to your mouth. Self-knowledge is a warning light that makes you less likely to react blindly or out of habit.

Conversely, insights can trip green lights. When you recognize a positive personality trait, such as taking a walk instead of snacking on sweets, you will get a "go" signal from your mind for this healthy behavior.

Many of us have used food to repress our signals, both positive and negative. Without excess food, we can use the tools of self-knowledge to lose pounds—permanently.

Members of diet groups have ample opportunity to share their insight, strength, and hope with each other without fear of embarrassment. In fact, your insight can turn a light on to another person's hidden problem, and vice versa.

Practice sharing insights with other overeaters. The more you share, the more you know yourself. And the more others know you, the less you will feel you have to hide your true self.

### The Life Preservers Around You

Food is our most available nonprescription tranquilizer. Does extra food make you feel good? If you're honest with yourself, you'll have to answer yes. But think about how long that good feeling lasts. It is fleeting at best. A few seconds of relief, of comfort, of tasting something sweet seem a small reward compared to the high price you pay for it.

In the past, you got a quick fix from food. What other sources can you use now to relieve anxiety? Begin by finding someone you can talk to about your feelings of dis-ease. You may find that your anxieties are really false fears that dissipate as you talk about them. But even if they are real, you cut their power over you in half by sharing them.

Most people who have lost weight have had the help and support of an understanding friend—be it wife, husband, fellow dieter, a good listener. Try to identify the most sympathetic friend or relative you know, someone who loves you in moments of failure as well as success. When you feel an almost uncontrollable urge to grab the unhealthiest food you can reach, contact that person. Ask this person if he or she would help you kick a tough habit. Explain that you are taking off weight one day at a time and may need some help occasionally.

Reassure your friend that this won't be a full-time job. It might mean simply lending an ear in times of stress—times when you're tempted to side-step a problem by eating unneeded food. Setting up this arrangement is like creating a safety net. You now have someone to call when you feel an almost uncontrollable urge to grab the unhealthiest food you can reach. You know that someone who approves of your efforts is ready to listen and help you.

Compulsive eaters are essentially lonely people. Overeating takes time, energy, and concentration, plus lots of time alone. We don't want others watching an act that we, ourselves, find disgusting. Perhaps we eat to gratify a need for human contact. But we find it difficult to relate to people because we're afraid of being hurt. For good reason, we don't see people as particularly friendly.

If you feel this deep loneliness, you may want to seek out people like yourself who are working toward a common goal. You'll find immediate acceptance among such people. Consider joining a support group for overeaters, or at least visit one. Loneliness is a misery you don't have to feel.

One reason we suffer loneliness is that we're hiding the guilty secret of our behavior. We think we're the only one in the world who ever ate candy bars in the bathroom and hid the wrappers in the clothes hamper. Joining a support group soon enlightens us. We discover that we are not alone—others kept such eating secrets too, and these secrets can only be shared with others in the same boat.

In a support group, you'll get a sense of relief at having friends around who understand what you're going through, friends who have been there. You won't need to pretend for them. You won't have to show them how "right" everything is with you.

You will discover other people with eating problems, sometimes far worse than yours. This identification is essential to an increased feeling of well-being. You are no longer alone. And to an overeater, this is one of the greatest feelings in the world.

You'll also learn to accept help. In a support group, you'll find people in various stages of recovery who are willing to freely give you the same help that was given to them.

Finally, as you begin to overcome your own eating problems, you will be able to help newcomers. You will be a mentor where before you could scarcely help yourself.

Sure, everyone wants to appear strong and self-reliant, but if you're drowning in a sea of food, grab for a life preserver. A group can help rescue you for several reasons:

1. Allies, though they may have an overeating problem greater than yours, have strengths from which you can benefit.

2. You need others to share your enthusiasm. And when you're down, you need the enthusiasm of others to help lift you up again.

3. Other recovering overeaters will refuse to verify your negative self-image, helping you gain fresh insights.

4. Success is attractive. The success of others will spur you on, and your own success will help others. Both are great affirmations of your new way of food-controlled living.

5. Other people help motivate you to keep your promises. When you tell yourself and others what you intend to do, you are apt to keep that commitment.

6. A support group helps expand your value system; you learn from the goodness of others.

You can best help others and yourself by being truthful and positive when sharing your insights and feelings. That way, you'll receive what you truly need—honest support.

When you share feelings, don't blame others (e.g., mom, dad, wife, husband, children, boss) for them. Own your feelings and communicate your weaknesses as well as your strengths.

If you only communicate what is comfortable, phoniness will establish distance between you and others.

Most important, learn to listen. Don't be so busy thinking of what to say next that you miss others' contributions.

The most helpful insights often come from other people. This means we can't always be filling the air with our own words. We have to let silence work for us now and then. We also have to give others time to respond to our feelings.

## Reaching Beyond Your Inner Circle

Once you've found your peers in the safety of a support group, you can apply your sharing and understanding skills to outsiders as well. Now you can open yourself to new experiences by seeking similarities in nondieters. But be prepared for a shock. Slender people have living problems similar to our own. Overweight people often have a Cinderella complex: we tend to think that when we are thin, we won't have any problems. This is simply not true.

A good plan is to relate to other overweight people for your weight problem, but for the remainder of your living experience, relate to everyone you meet—overweight and thin alike. We often divide the world into fat and thin. But this world is much more diverse, and we can find similarities with others very different from us. So it is entirely possible for you to find that you have a good deal in common with a wide variety of people, regardless of their weight.

However, finding common ground will take some work on your part. It's easy, after all, to see differences: "Oh, she's not fat; what could she know?" It's true that thinner people may not be able to help us with our weight problem, but they can give us examples of their courage, strength, friendship, and faith.

Try not to see yourself as lonely and misunderstood. Take a look around to see ways in which all humans are alike. Deliberately seeking similarities, you'll find, is a positive approach to your new way of living without excess food.

We can train ourselves to become more receptive to the wisdom of others by doing the following:

1. Seek out positive qualities in others.

2. Transcend negative feelings about other people by going out of your way to help them.

3. Don't attach conditions to the help you give.

4. Realize that the faults you recognize in other people are really the faults that you unconsciously hate in yourself.

5. Find something in others to praise.

6. Learn to recognize times when someone needs your support but is unable to ask for it.

7. Support others without subordinating your own values or needs.

Most important, remember every single day that you are reaching for a weight that is healthy for you. And you can achieve your goal if you develop emotional stability and a strong support structure. You must let others contribute to your well-being, while you contribute to theirs.

It's as simple as it sounds. You are taking responsibility for your own behavior and you are aware of how your behavior affects others. That makes you a strong person and, ultimately, a thin person.

Some overweight people have spent a lifetime proving to others and to themselves that they can't "take it." Like a fragile Christmas gift, some of us come wrapped with the words *Handle with Care* stamped all over us.

We *are* sensitive people. But some of us have become very good at playing the wounded martyr. We see nonexistent slights and we sulk over imaginary insults. After a while, we stop attracting the attention and concern we're longing for, so we escalate the emotional displays. Sometimes, we substitute sympathy and pity—our own and other people's—for love. Don't confuse sympathy with positive help. If you are eating right for health and weight loss, you won't need negative attention. As you grow away from your addiction to excess food, you will become strong enough to withstand emotional discomfort. As your confidence builds, a new person will emerge, one who does not need the feeling of pity—indeed, one who rejects it.

The important thing to remember through all change is that, as you change, you are creating your life anew. A yoga master once said: "Begin to know that creation is merely recognizing what is already there—that there is nothing new; everything is within you and is portrayed on the outside as you become aware that it is already created, finished, within you."

*Everything is within you.* All the things you want to be, you already are. All the things you want to have, you already have.

Now that you know this truth, you have expanded your self-awareness. Your new sense of awareness lets you focus on what is real. And when you focus your awareness on what you truly are inside, you can project it outside yourself.

A Sanskrit proverb begins: "Look to this day, for it is life, the very life of life. Become aware, today, of all that you are, for only then will you know what you can create out of this day."

You can begin the creation of a new life during the

next twenty-four hours. In order to match your outside to your inside, you must begin to bring order to your eating, to your thinking, and to your feeling. When you do, you will quiet the conflict excess food has created.

# CHAPTER 4

# Positive Doing

## Changing Your Old Habits

*Y*ou are on a quest to become your best. No longer powerless, you have accepted responsibility for yourself and have begun to implement health-supporting behavior into your daily routines. First, you learned how your negative thoughts and feelings piled on the pounds; then you discovered how positive power made your life work better. Now, it's time to take action that will help you gain mastery over your food desires and get your body moving. It's time to permanently change your eating and exercise habits.

If you don't have a personal eating plan for healthy weight loss, construct one now, specifically for yourself. No one else has your particular weight history, body type, physical needs, food preferences, or family life. You're unique. A weight group plan or published diet may be right for you, but if you don't find one ready-made, do your research and customize your own. "Personal" diets are often the most successful.

In this chapter, you'll find some basic nutrition information to get you started, but remember that this isn't a nutrition book. You'll need to get further information from your doctor, your library, or the resources listed in the back of this book. And you'll find that when you begin to lose weight for your good health, you'll naturally become more interested in learning how to do it better.

Prepare to revise your eating plan as you go along. Change is good. We need to continually learn and make adjustments in every area of our lives and in our way of eating most of all.

The same goes for your personal exercise plan. Pat yourself on the back for what you're already doing, even if it's walking up stairs instead of taking the elevator, then determine to do more. Begin with activities that are fun for you or that look like fun. Then go for it. If you're over forty, don't let your age stop you. As fitness coach and author Joan Price says, "You're not over the hill, you're on top of it."

Sometimes, after years of being sedentary and feeling negative about our bodies, we are ashamed to exercise in public. We think we would rather die than put on a swimsuit. But don't use shame as an excuse for inaction; use your newfound self-acceptance as a key to living more happily in your body.

No one is telling you to grab some bottled water, put on a sweatband and jump into an intense step aerobics class, unless that is what you want to do. You can make an easier start. For example, the least expensive and most available exercise in the world is right outside your door—walking. Walk with a friend or try mall-walking with an organized group.

Gradually refine and add variety to your personal exercise plan. Make your start and then continue to build exercise routines into each day until you have the healthy, functioning body you want. Experts tell us that it's better to add time rather than intensity to our workout. The longer you exercise, the more you burn fat from your fat stores, and that's what you're after.

Exercise helps your body repair and improve itself to an amazing degree. It strengthens your heart and lungs, lowers your blood pressure, builds and tones your muscles, and keeps your joints and tendons more flexible. If that's not enough, add to the list increased energy, improved sleep, and reduced tension. It may even extend your life. Exercise is looking more like an ordinary act that gives you extraordinary results.

You don't *have* to exercise in order to lose weight, but it speeds up weight loss, improves your metabolism, suppresses your appetite, and speeds you through weight plateaus. Calories continue to burn even after exercise. Plus, exercise contributes to your overall health and enhances your self-esteem.

When you begin to change the destructive eating and exercise habits of a lifetime, your old negative self may try to convince you that you're being punished. But your new positive self knows better. You just need time to achieve solid benefits. Give yourself that time. The rewards will come.

### Take a Reality Check

The first step in "Positive Doing" is making an honest assessment of yourself, identifying the old eating patterns that made you fat and kept you fat. Ask yourself the following three questions:

1. Do you use food to cushion your life against stress, taking the all-too-familiar escape route of overeating?

2. Have you identified trigger mechanisms—anger, self-pity, low energy—that set off your addictive responses to food?

3. Do you avoid people and situations that set you off on eating binges?

Remember, food offered the *illusion of escape.* Overeating only seemed to provide a remedy for your problems. But the reality was that excess food became your addiction, your uncontrolled eating a chronic, crippling disease.

To move forward in our weight-losing plan, we need to develop a sense of reality. We must deal realistically with the consequences of our overeating. In order to successfully bring our eating under control, we must learn to think of consequences *before* we eat, not after.

Recovery for us requires a complete reversal of old eating patterns. We must get a "new religion." Eating for weight loss and eventual health maintenance must be paramount. Our born-again bodies must be so important to us that we'll do anything to keep them.

You used to think you could take just one bite and stop; now you know that's not true. What you need now is a warning bell that goes off in your head *before* you ever start the awful bite-after-bite binge. What you need now is self-control. Self-control is really personal courage. It tells you that you can endure, and it's the way you maintain confidence in yourself. With self-control, you will believe in yourself and in your abilities.

For the overeater, self-control comes down to resisting the first bite of unneeded food. As Benjamin Franklin said, "It is easier to suppress the first desire than to satisfy all that follow it." That first extra bite is easier to stop than the binge that can follow. For today, refuse that first bite of food not on your eating plan. You'll find that self-control is nothing more or less than an ongoing, never-ending series of healthy choices.

And if your self-control does start to slip, it's reassuring to know that you are equipped with safety controls: two sets of powerful eating brakes. *Basic brakes* can stop a food accident on a dime before it ever happens. *Emergency brakes* applied quickly can bring an eating skid to a screeching halt after it starts.

One of the best basic brakes is a vivid mental image of yourself looking the way you want to look. By programming your mind with positive self-imagery, you can invoke this image when you need it most. And if you do this often enough, you will develop a healthy, new eating control.

If you've already taken that first bite, apply your emergency brake with a loud "No!" when you reach for the next bite. Better yet, spit out the first one. This is a powerful act your mind will remember.

Repetition can also become discipline—the trait most of us can use in abundance. To de-emphasize food, some dieters try to eat the same things every day. This repetition appears to relieve them of their former preoccupation with food, its preparation, and menu decisions. Dr. John McDougall notes in his book *The McDougall Program for Maximum Weight Loss:* "More is eaten during a meal consisting of a variety of foods than during a meal with just one food, even if that food is a favorite."

Leading a more structured life will open up time for upgrading your self-image. Use that time to recall your past successes. See yourself forming positive new habits and dropping worn-out negative ones. Find pleasure in the simple, structured rhythm of your life.

### We Are Different

According to Dr. Richard B. Stuart, six things distinguish us overeaters from people who have always been thin.

1. *Overweight people eat more food when it is readily available.* That means we tend to eat less if inconvenience or work is required to obtain the food. How can you make problem foods less available to you?

2. *Overweight people are triggered to eat more food*

*whenever they see and smell it.* Thin people usually get hungry on a time basis—from four to six hours after eating a meal. What can you do to remove food from your sight and smell between regular meals?

3. *Taste is more important to overweight people.* When groups of thin and fat people had unlimited access to unpalatable foods, the overweight group tended to eat less. How can you limit your choices of favorite foods?

4. *Overweight people eat until there is no more food on their plate or table;* thin people stop eating when they feel full. Can you limit the portions on your plate and remove extra food from the table in advance?

5. *Overweight people seem to be less aware of the caloric and nutritional value of foods they eat.* How can you learn more about the nutritional content of the foods you eat?

6. *Overweight people get less exercise than thin people.* How can you increase the amount of exercise you get?

Researchers have made other observations on the eating patterns of thin people:

Thinner eaters take fewer bites per minute and take smaller bites. They have more noneating responses, such as playing with food, hesitating, putting their utensil down, drinking between bites. After eating, thinner eaters also depart from the table sooner, are rated less tense, and leave more food on their plates.

The results of these observations are obvious, but they bear repeating for emphasis: *Thin people do eat differently.*

What does this data mean for you? Simply, if you imitate the way thin people eat, you are more likely to weigh what they weigh.

*Recognizing Destructive Habits*

Recognizing poor eating habits and putting an end to

them is how we begin making the switch from destructive eating to "Positive Doing."

*Snack Sneaking*

"I never eat a whole meal," a very overweight woman told her doctor. "I can't imagine how I gained so much weight." This woman was really suffering from an affliction that attacks many overeaters—snack sneaking. She ate a mouthful here, a bite there. While serving a meal to her family, she "tasted" all of it to make certain it was properly spiced and heated. She "didn't have time" to sit down and eat a full meal, so she grabbed and snatched food all day long, kidding herself all the time that she wasn't eating much at all.

The doctor told her that, instead of eating her usual bite, taste, or piece of food, she should put it in a container. "I only did it for part of one day," the woman later admitted. "I was shocked when I ended up with an enormous bowl of food." Like other snack sneakers, she lost weight rapidly once she changed her eating pattern to three meals a day—consumed only at a table.

All of us can be great self-deceivers. We can cover up the worst eating habits by just *not paying attention*.

We also play conscious tricks to cover up our unhealthy habits. "I hid candy," said one dieter at a group meeting. "I put it under my clothes, on the shelf of my linen closet, even in the bathroom. And then I hid myself away so that I could eat it without being caught.

"I became so good at eating undiscovered, nobody could understand how I gained so much weight, since I hardly ate a thing in front of people."

The Institute of Human Nutrition recently estimated that overweight people eat as much as half of their food *away* from the table. It's apparent that secret eating habits must be broken to achieve weight loss. "I tell my patients to sit down for a moment and ask themselves, 'Am I hungry?' not 'Do I want to eat it?'" says Dr. Barbara Felland. "The answer is usually, 'No, I'm not hungry.'"

Constant snacking is as hard on the discipline you're trying to build as it is on your figure. Say no to your small food demands and you'll be able to say no to the big binges when you're tempted. A disciplined way of eating for health and thinness is built on saying no to a return to destructive old habits.

*Idle Eating*

Chances are, if you're doing a lot of snack sneaking, you're not busy enough. Snacking is often done to relieve boredom or tension.

The solution is to keep busy. How many tasks have you left undone because you thought you were too fat to accomplish them? Do them today, or at least make a good beginning. Try some new activities, such as hiking, biking, or the hobby you've always wanted to try.

Of course, it's also possible to become a compulsive worker. Since overeaters often tend toward over-everything, we have to be especially careful that we don't use work to make up for our physical shortcomings. Then, too, it is possible to overwork until we convince ourselves that we need *extra* food just to keep going.

Moderating our activity is as important as moderating our food intake. Too much or too little—both can contribute to our eating problem.

But don't confuse resting with idling. Rest is necessary. It's the pause that refreshes our bodies and our spirits.

Food, work, rest—all in proper proportion—bring balance and harmony into your life. What a marvelous new experience.

*Speed Eating*

Studies show (and we know it ourselves) that overeaters are compulsive about the quantity of food they eat and the frequency with which they eat it. We are also fast eaters. We can wolf down meals long before others are finished.

If you are overweight, you are probably not a slow, leisurely eater, but such rapid-fire eating can be slowed down. Dab your mouth with a napkin, make conversation, or sip water rather than taking one automatic bite after another. Behaviorists call this delaying technique "chaining." It simply means that you are linking together noneating behavior.

Psychiatrists Walter H. Fanburg and Bernard M. Snyder offer six other suggestions to help us eat more slowly. These techniques give our stomachs time to signal our brain that we're not hungry anymore.

1. Do not pick up another bite of food until you have chewed and swallowed the one in your mouth.

2. Take a rest period after a certain number of mouthfuls (three, for example).

3. Put your fork down frequently.

4. Pay more attention to the taste, smell, and texture of food.

5. Try to be the last person to finish each course of a meal.

6. Never finish a meal in less than twenty minutes.

If you are a "grab-and-eat" person, slow down. Remove food from its container. Carry it to the table. Get out utensils and plates. Sit down at the table. All these actions act as buffers between your desire for food and the act of eating. Adopt these rituals and you'll be able to concentrate on the good eating habits you're trying to form.

*Crash Dieting*

There's another way speed can wreck your diet. If you are a "results now" person, learn to be patient and steady when it comes to your weight loss. Crash diets only cause crashes.

We all want to hurry up and get off those pounds. But don't push toward your goal at an unsafe speed. It's inconsistent with the positive restructuring of your life. Overaccelerating is bound to lead to faulty judgment. "I'll skip breakfast today," you say; or, "I'll fast for a week," hoping to step up the weight-loss process. Most likely, you won't. You'll get too hungry or too weak.

Instead, select a target weight and commit yourself to reach that goal. (You may want to work with your doctor to determine your *natural* weight and set that as your goal or you may want to choose the weight where you looked and felt the best. Every person, regardless of height and sex, has a unique natural weight. Height-and-weight charts are rarely useful.) That's the important first step. Equally important is selecting the method or plan you intend to use and then committing yourself to this method. If you are finding your own way—the method that regulates your diet and weight loss—then you won't fall victim to the hurry-up syndrome. What's more, you'll probably enjoy the weight-loss process more. Each day will bring fresh insights. You'll be learning about yourself, so that when you reach your natural weight you'll have new confidence.

For most of us, a healthy way of eating plus exercise and re-ordered mental priorities remain the only realistic way to take off weight permanently and safely. Regaining lost weight is a devastating experience, so commit yourself to a weight goal and a plan to reach that goal today.

*Changing Old Patterns*

If you've had the overeating habit for some time, you need to be "reprogrammed." You need to develop some new, weight-losing habits. Behavior contributes to weight problems. When we recognize negative behaviors and commit to changing them, we will begin to develop the eating habits that will lead us to a thinner life.

*Slow It Down, Turn It Around*

Eat nutritious food in a calm and slow manner. Allow your meals to become a part of your day, but not its whole focus.

You can do this by literally watching how you eat. Take a portable mirror to the table and watch yourself closely. While eating, try to observe as many details as you can: bite size, appearance of mouth and cheeks, and how quickly you finish your food. This exercise can make you more conscious of your eating pattern and help you to develop slower, more rational, and more orderly habits.

Watching *how much* you eat and *when* can also be beneficial to weight loss. It has been found that Americans eat most of their food *after* 6 p.m. Unfortunately, they get little or no exercise after the biggest meal of the day. The next morning, it's easy to skip breakfast; lunch is a normal-sized meal, and dinner is again huge.

Try turning your eating upside down. Make your most substantial meal breakfast, and reduce your intake throughout the day. Your good sense tells you that you will burn more food as energy and lose more weight. Dieters who reverse their eating habits also have a better disposition, are less tired, more productive, and in better control of emotions as the day wears on.

Some weight-loss programs help members adopt healthier habits by suggesting they follow behavior modification techniques, phased in over a period of time:

The first week, practice sitting down while eating, plus using the proper utensils. (If you eat at your desk at work, clear your desk and set a place as you would your dining table.)

The second week, practice eating with no distractions—no reading, radio, or TV. This will help you concentrate *only* on your eating.

The third week, adopt a slower eating style.

The fourth week, write your daily menu (including any snacks allowed) in advance. This halts spontaneous eating.

The fifth week, put some time between your desire to eat and the act of eating itself.

The sixth week calls for a discipline overeaters rarely practice: Leave some food on your plate. This shows that you have control over food; food doesn't have control over you.

It is helpful to be aware of the way you *act* when food is around and of the unconscious *cues* that prompt you to eat more. Most weight-loss programs suggest some form of self-monitoring, for example, by writing down everything you eat during a day, where you eat, and your emotional state at the time. You are more likely to overeat at certain times and places, and when in certain moods—and not even be aware of the pattern. A written record gives you insight into your unconscious eating behavior.

Why is awareness so important in successful dieting? Because it tends to break up the habit of eating indiscriminately. Awareness adds another dimension to your response to food—thinking.

*Out of Sight, Out of Mind—and Body*

It's only good sense to keep tempting foods out of your way. Most diet experts suggest you purge your pantry of all "goodies"—you can't eat them if you don't have them. Conversely, keep on hand the good, healthy foods that your personal eating plan calls for. Without the right stuff in the house, you can't eat properly, either.

Another helpful thing you can do for yourself is to keep food out of sight. You can do it even while cooking: take a single ingredient from the cupboard or refrigerator, and return it before you take out another. Avoid high-calorie convenience foods that lend themselves to snacking; choose instead simple dishes that require fresh, whole ingredients.

Being overwhelmed while preparing meals is one problem, but another is shopping for food. The ancient Roman warning "Let the buyer beware!" goes double for dieters in today's supermarkets. Stores are filled with a dizzying variety and quantity of foods, all attractively packaged and within easy reach. As you walk down the aisle, you pass hundreds of food items per minute. It's no wonder that many shoppers use the grab-and-snatch method of food selection.

Before you head for the store, make a list of healthy foods on your eating plan, shop only from that list, and bring only enough cash to cover that list. You won't be as likely to pick up junk foods if you plan ahead.

Here's another important tip: do your shopping after you've eaten—hungry people buy more food. Transport your newly purchased groceries in the trunk rather than on the car seat next to you. Billions of calories have been consumed between supermarket parking lots and people's homes.

When choosing foods for purchase, stop to read the

package labels. This might slow down your shopping a bit, but you will know exactly what you're putting into your body. By law, all ingredients must be listed in the order of predominance. That means if fat or sugar in any form is listed above the third ingredient, this product probably shouldn't be on your weight-losing diet.

Labels also spell out the nutrient value of food, gram by gram. They give the amount of fat, sugar, protein, and carbohydrates. Practice some simple arithmetic. Multiply the grams of sugar, protein, and carbohydrates by four and the fat grams by nine to get the calorie count of each, then divide each into the total number of calories per serving to get their percentage. For example, if you are watching your fat intake and want to keep it under 20 percent, don't buy a product with a calorie count of 100 calories per cup if it contains 5 grams of fat. At 9 calories per gram of fat, the product would contain 45 percent fat per serving, far above the level you want to maintain.

Try to organize your schedule so that you do all your grocery shopping in one trip each week. Careful planning can eliminate the need to keep going back every other day—the more trips you make to the store, the more likely you are to buy impulse, fattening food on one of the trips. (If some items won't keep for a week, let someone else go to the store.)

Once you get your groceries home and cooked, don't store your leftovers in plain sight, creating a tempting display of potential snacks every time you open your refrigerator. Pack them in nontransparent plastic containers. This builds a delay between wanting and actually getting to the food you don't need.

*Build Awareness*
Members of diet support groups often claim they

overeat without realizing it. "I finished the whole box of candy," one person complained, "and didn't remember picking it up. I just sort-of 'came to' with it in my hand."

It's true that some overeaters are not conscious of their overeating habits. Through repetition, these habits become so routine that a dieter must deliberately place something between the thought and the act of eating.

To zap old eating patterns and alert yourself to what you are doing, try some awareness-jogging tricks. Place reminders of your new eating program on refrigerator doors and kitchen cabinets. Don't eat while you are doing something else—watching television, for example. While you are engrossed in the action, eating becomes automatic, one bite following another.

Kicking old eating habits is an indispensable element of successful dieting. It may seem a bit childish to write down daily menus or paste diet program slogans all over the kitchen, but that may be where you have to start—at the beginning.

Here are some guidelines to keep in mind when making the change to new, positive eating habits:

1. *Re-educate your eyes by measuring your food.* Learn precisely what a cup of food looks like to ensure correct portions.

2. *Never skip a meal.* It's not the way to lose weight faster. Chances are you'll just get so hungry you will eat more than twice as much at the next meal.

3. *Talk yourself out of unscheduled snacks.* Set a kitchen timer for ten minutes and relax. Lie down or do some simple meditation exercises. When the timer rings, you will realize you are not that hungry after all.

4. *Ask yourself "how" instead of "why" questions.* For example, don't ask, "Why can't I ever stay on a diet?" Ask instead, "How can I stay with my weight-losing plan?"

5. *Don't let yourself eat the whole thing.* If you slip and start eating a piece of a high-calorie treat—stop before you've polished off the entire piece.

6. *Plan for success.* Be on the lookout for new tips and ideas that might work to help you lose weight.

7. *Lead a less food-oriented life.* Do everything possible to divert your attention from food and the mythical pleasures of eating.

### Dieting in All the Wrong Places

"I got so excited at the ball game," said one dieter to his doctor, "that when it was over I found myself sitting with two empty beer cans, a hot dog wrapper, and a pile of peanut shells."

Eating, for many of us, becomes so automatic during certain occasions that we give little thought to what is being eaten. Traditional (but destructive) eating habits can easily surface during athletic events, television watching, vacations, and holidays. These situations give us an excuse to indulge—to fall into the old patterns we've been working so hard to change.

Nevertheless, it's extremely difficult to eat without having some awareness. The alibi "It's the Super Bowl, after all. *Everyone* overeats at Super Bowl parties" is an attempt to take responsibility away from ourselves and place blame on the occasion.

One solution would be to avoid the occasion altogether, or to go for a walk instead of taking part in the activity that prompts you to overeat. But often, especially on holidays, the occasion cannot be avoided. A better solution is to recognize your destructive behavior patterns and take the responsibility to sidestep them.

If formal dining is your weakness, the following tips can help you in a restaurant, at a party, at a holiday dinner, or in any other situation where the main focus is on food.

1. Choose low-calorie and low-fat menu items when eating out. Try eating a salad as an entree, skipping fat-filled dressings and other ingredients. Always ask for dressings on the side so that you can control the amount. Go ahead and have the whole-grain roll; just skip the butter.

2. Avoid drinking alcohol with your meal. Make water your main beverage. Bottled water with a slice of lemon or lime can be quite satisfying.

3. Drink water or diet soda before your meal, and eat your meal slowly.

4. Focus on the event not your food. Enjoy the conversation and company of others.

With forethought, you can confidently step over the pitfalls of overeating. You can avoid the vicious cycle of overeating out of frustration, boredom, and lack of planning, and then overeating even more, *because* you are frustrated, bored, and lack a well-defined plan. The way to get off that destructive merry-go-round is to break the cycle of overeating—today and forever.

## It's All in Your Head

In addition to unhealthy eating patterns, subtle psychological and emotional factors can trick us into eating over our feelings. We must build defenses against these less-apparent factors if we are to turn our food habits in a new and healthier direction.

### Eating for Security

Behavioral psychologists maintain that patterns are the culprits in the war against fat. They recommend that we discover our patterns (habits) relating to certain foods, places, times, and feelings.

Many of us associate a certain taste with a pleasant, secure memory. When we're depressed, we try to reproduce these feelings by eating these memory foods. By overeating these foods, we may be subconsciously attempting to recapture the safety of childhood or another time when we felt especially secure.

To overeaters, food is often more than food. Like overzealous mothers, we use it to reward or punish ourselves. But in order to lose our excess weight and keep it off, we must learn that food is not more than food—it is not love—it is just food.

Some of us also turn in the opposite direction and think of food as an enemy. But food is not an enemy, either; it is just food—fuel for life.

Building a healthier relationship with food begins with being willing to recognize areas in your life where you resist growing up. All of us make excuses that seem plausible. But in no area do we have more excuses than for our eating behavior. "I need this food because I'm (tired, sick, unloved, nervous, anxious, rejected, frightened, or any number of other feelings.)"

A need for security can affect our eating in other ways. Many overweight people, particularly those who have been fat since childhood, have a hidden fear of becoming thin. They think they dare not risk unfamiliar feelings, places, or people. When psychologists ask them what they fear most about being thin, many name a loss of security. Said one obese man, "My security is knowing how to act. I only know how to act fat."

Overeaters' insecurities can be sex-related. Some overweight people fear promiscuity should they suddenly become more desirable. "There is a vivacious, slim woman deep inside me," said one married woman, almost sixty pounds overweight. "How would this other 'me' handle a pass from an attractive man? I feel safer when I'm fat because nobody wants me, so I never have to worry about breaking my marriage vows."

There is little worth striving for that does not carry

risk. Becoming slender after a period of being over-weight will alter your lifestyle considerably. You'll go through a period of adjustment. Being thin doesn't mean that you will have no problems. But if you have concentrated on really getting to know yourself, you will have developed resources to deal with whatever you encounter.

*Eating for Approval*

When you were a child, your teachers may have returned your outstanding papers with smiley faces or "Good Work" stickers on top. Sometimes, after a series of awards, you could look forward to an extra treat—usually something sweet—for being such a good boy or girl.

Some of us adults still give ourselves treats. Take the experience of one dieter: "At a family dinner, I firmly stuck to my eating plan," she reported. "Everyone admired my willpower as I turned down one fattening dessert after another.

"I felt really good about myself. Then I got home, and before I knew it, I had eaten almost every sweet thing in my refrigerator—much more than I'd turned down at the dinner. Why did I do that?"

The answer? This dieter, like so many, is a member of the "good boy/girl" club. We reward ourselves with smiley faces for turning in a good dieting performance, and when we accumulate enough stars, we turn them in for a binge.

This syndrome is so ingrained that we experience it repeatedly without understanding the subtle game we're playing. Indeed, we are so confused by our behavior that we begin to doubt our intelligence, if not our sanity. The root of this mystifying syndrome lies in our need for approval.

Nobody can go through life without occasionally needing the approval of others. But problems occur when we constantly need others to tell us we are capable, intelligent, good, or even thin enough. The truth is, we don't really seek honest evaluations; we seek agreement. When we don't get it, our whole day can be ruined, and as a result we can overeat.

Some of us choose a path that seems to guarantee a continuous stream of approval from others. We try in every way to please others. Of course, this generally means we are false to ourselves. Our aim is to *prevent any chance of rejection.*

But you can't please all of the people all of the time. You need to think more about pleasing yourself. Although it may seem a contradiction, you will find that the more you please yourself, the more independent you will become and the more others will be pleased.

*Eating for Others*

Sometimes we take on the problems and failures of family, friends, and co-workers until the burden is too great to bear. Have you ever overeaten because others didn't do as you thought they should? When we spend so much time living through other people, we may be avoiding our own problems. Peace of mind comes only after we let go of any desire to "manage."

It's important to recognize that the responsibility for our problems is ours alone. If you do a good job of living your life, it will take all the energy and time you have. You must find a balance between living with others and not living so closely that you invade their sphere of responsibility. That does not mean you should ignore them. It means that you should *tend to your own needs first.* Ultimately *you are responsible* for your behavior.

Don't be surprised if you find something about this

thought with which to argue. It's a disquieting notion that the behavior of others can't influence us unless we let it. But ridding yourself of the right to blame other people puts you in charge of your own life. Now you are free from the ill will of people or the circumstance of birth. Whatever has gone before, you are in control today.

By being committed to self-responsibility, you are proving that attitude is vital to successful weight loss. Positive attitudes are earmarks of those who graduate into the healthy thin world. How many of these seven success attitudes can you actively use in your life?

1. *Honesty*—Freedom from self-deception and sneak-eating.

2. *Willingness*—Ability to admit a mistake, take firm steps to correct a diet error, and deal fairly with yourself.

3. *Courage*—Dealing with problems and realities of life without relying on extra snacks to "pull you through"; determination to stick to it no matter how insistently your body cries out for more food.

4. *Appreciation*—Gratitude for a healthy mental attitude, the one that urges you to change your life.

5. *Openmindedness*—Receptiveness to suggestions that help you live without excess food and build a positive new lifestyle.

6. *Humility*—Ability to face facts, to recognize that you have lost control of your eating, and to see that you are not too proud to accept help.

7. *Service*—Repaying the help you received by passing it on to other dieters whenever possible.

Take a close look at this checklist; you won't find time- or money-consuming demands on it. Try to acquire these success attitudes. You have much to gain in positive attitudes, and you'll lose weight.

*From Here to Serenity*

The Serenity Prayer is spoken in dozens of languages daily by millions of people throughout the world. The point of the prayer is simply the desire to see things clearly and realistically. It is both spiritual in nature and very practical:

> *God, grant me the serenity*
> *to accept the things I cannot change,*
> *the courage to change the things I can,*
> *and the wisdom to know the difference.*

The Serenity Prayer is a perfect antidote to negativity. By repeating these words, many overeaters find it possible to cope with feelings of frustration, anger, and aggression. They often find the comfort in those words allows them to replace negative, destructive feelings with positive, constructive actions.

The word *serenity* used here is not a nothingness, but a stillness within. Too many overweight people conduct ceaseless self-questioning about what, when, why, and how they are overeating. Our struggle with food keeps us in turmoil. What we need is the stillness of serenity.

When you face a problem, ask yourself: Is this a problem I can solve? Can I take action today? If so, what action? If you make a decision to act, do so. If you decide that action is unwise, do nothing. Vacillation only leads to food binges. From here on, guard your serenity; make decisions based on constructive thinking.

Learning to live a day at a time is one of the most positive things compulsive people can do for themselves. Whether we're addicted to food, alcohol, or to some other drug, our big problem is dealing with the present.

One of the favorite whips with which we overeaters flog ourselves is the lament over a wasted past. "If only I had started my weight-losing program when I was younger!" we cry. Unable to change the past, we sometimes sink into depression and overeat more. "What's the use? I'll soon be forty (or fifty or sixty) and my youth will be over for good." Of course, it seldom occurs to us that we'll be forty in any event, and that it's our choice whether we'll be forty and fat or forty and thin.

When not agonizing over a wasted youth, we worry about the future. Too often we visualize gloom and failure. "Next year will just be more of the same; I'll always be fat." But this future won't happen if you take care of today.

## Get Healthy with Good Nutrition

Even the most conscientious physician can't help us if we don't practice self-help. The first, most obvious move we can make is to eat a healthy diet. To do this— as we saw earlier in this chapter—most of us must take a hard look at our destructive eating habits, let them go one by one, and replace them with healthy habits. Our next step is to learn about nutrition—what food does to our bodies.

Many of us are professional dieters—we've been on about every diet ever invented. As a result, we tend to think we know everything about nutrition. In some ways we do. It's not possible to be as focused on food and eating as we are without learning the basics. For instance, most of us know that we gain more weight eating chocolates than rutabagas. Nonetheless, we may not be as nutrition-wise as we think we are. Few of us eat a truly healthful diet, containing proper proportions of fats, carbohydrates, and proteins together with necessary vitamins and minerals.

If you have doubts about the nutritional balance of your eating plan to lose or maintain your natural weight, consult a doctor or professional nutritionist.

But to be truly in control, you will need to discover food facts for yourself. Only then will you be able to drop cherished, but erroneous, ideas about the food you eat. Make it your business to learn more about nutrition. Learn how much protein your body really needs, which vegetables contain high concentrations of essential vitamins and minerals, what foods supply enough fiber to compensate for today's overprocessed foods.

This information is no secret. State health departments, the federal government, and a number of books supply information to help you choose the healthiest foods. (Some recommended books can be found on page 451.) Another good reference, shown here, is the U.S. Department of Agriculture's food pyramid, which has replaced the four basic food groups as a guide to recommended daily servings of types of food.

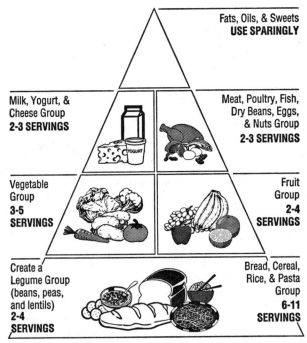

Fats, Oils, & Sweets
**USE SPARINGLY**

Milk, Yogurt, & Cheese Group
**2-3 SERVINGS**

Meat, Poultry, Fish, Dry Beans, Eggs, & Nuts Group
**2-3 SERVINGS**

Vegetable Group
**3-5 SERVINGS**

Fruit Group
**2-4 SERVINGS**

Create a Legume Group (beans, peas, and lentils)
**2-4 SERVINGS**

Bread, Cereal, Rice, & Pasta Group
**6-11 SERVINGS**

Source: U.S. Department of Agriculture

You owe it to yourself to discover the truth about what you eat. You should know what each food does for your weight loss or maintenance, and for your health. This is one of the duties of a responsible person who plans to enjoy maximum living.

### Begin with the Basics

Don't be overwhelmed by the number of foods and facts to learn. Your main task is clear. It's about choosing foods that will do the best for your body. You can start learning now with these guidelines.

### Fat

The fat you eat is the fat you wear. A gram of fat packs over twice as many calories as a gram of protein or carbohydrate. And we're learning that our western high-fat diet is literally killing us.

The China-Cornell-Oxford project, directed by Cornell University's Dr. T. Colin Campbell and reported in a recent issue of *Eating Well,* showed that the less fat people consume, the thinner and healthier they are. Likewise, rates of obesity, heart disease, breast cancer, and colon cancer fall dramatically as fat consumption declines.

Since most people in western cultures—Europe and America—get 60 percent of their fat from meat and dairy products, that would seem to be the logical place to start cutting. Asian and Mediterranean diets, for instance, are centered on fresh vegetables and carbohydrates—rice and noodles for the Asians and tomatoes and pasta for the Mediterraneans.

A question arises: "For good health, doesn't one's diet need fat?" Yes, but very little. Actually, of your total nutritional intake, only about 7 percent needs to be fat. Anything over that amount could end up on your hips, breasts, abdomen, face, and upper arms.

A good start to reducing your fat intake would be to cut the fat in your diet in half. You don't have to make this reduction all at once. Over a period of several weeks or months you can replace half your meat- and dairy-centered meals with starch-centered meals based on breads, grains, beans, pasta, corn, and rice with vegetables and fruits on the side. When you must eat meat, use lean fish and poultry as *condiments*. If you have trouble picturing your plate without a hamburger, steak, or chop on it, imagine your favorite Asian restaurant and its dishes that use lots of rice, noodles, and vegetables, with small tiny strips of meat *for flavor.*

You can also reduce fat by trimming the visible fat from red meat, by eating skinless chicken, and by buying low-fat varieties of prepared meats and dairy products. Reducing your portions is another way to cut fat. A meat portion on most reasonable diets is considered to be three to four ounces (not the sixteen-ounce steak proudly advertised by your local steakhouse.)

Make it your business to learn about what types of dietary fat exist and what each does to your body.

Saturated fats are harsher on your health than unsaturated fats, but for losing weight, any fat consumed is fat that you'll wear.

How much fat is too much for you? Most experts say a weight-loss plan should contain no more than 20 percent fat. Here's how to convert this percentage into grams:

On a 1,500-calorie-a-day weight-losing diet, 20 percent of 1,500 equals 300 calories. Next, divide 300 by 9 (number of calories in each gram of fat.) You get 33.3 grams. Now keep a running total of the fat grams listed on all the foods you eat to make sure you don't go over the limit of 33.3 grams per day.

A plate of nachos and guacamole for lunch racks up 27 grams of fat, nearly your whole day's quota. But a big baked potato garnished with salsa, plus a generous salad with fat-free dressing registers close to zero grams. You make the choice.

*Protein*

The good news about protein is that you can eat twice as much of it (at 4 calories per gram) as fat (at 9 calories per gram) and still maintain the same calorie intake. The bad news is that you don't need nearly as much protein as you eat, and the excess could be harming you.

Many Americans worry about their protein intake, thinking they don't get enough. But, many of us actually suffer from excess protein consumption. A healthy male needs no more than 20 grams of protein a day, and yet consumes a daily average of 160 grams. What does your body do with the excess? Protein is not converted to fat or carbohydrate unless there is no carbohydrate available. And there's no place in your body to store the protein you don't use. So out it goes through your overworked kidneys, taking minerals, including calcium from your bones, with it. The loss of calcium can eventually lead to osteoporosis, a primary health concern for older women.

Most of our dietary protein comes from animals, so if you are already cutting back on saturated fat by substituting grains, pasta, potatoes, beans, and rice, you've automatically cut down on the excess protein that your body doesn't need.

Are you still worried about getting enough protein? According to the experts, you can actually live healthfully and lose weight on a diet that contains no more than 15 percent protein. Cornell's Dr. T. Colin Campbell reported that those living in rural China, who typically eat a rice-centered diet, live healthy, long lives on 6 percent protein. You probably don't need to cut your protein intake back that far, but you can easily cut back on your protein, lose weight, and gain health.

*Carbohydrates*

Carbohydrates could be a dieter's dream come true. Research shows that a diet rich in complex carbohydrates and low in fat seems to allow people to consume more calories without adding pounds.

Research at the Massachusetts Institute of Technology indicates that carbohydrate consumption increases the level of serotonin in the brain, a substance that boosts a person's sense of well-being. That could explain why we feel a momentary lift after eating a candy bar. Sugar is a carbohydrate, after all, but unfortunately for dieters, it usually comes wrapped in saturated fat in the form of chocolate or pastry. Carbohydrates from healthier sources will give you the same feeling of well-being with no awful rebound on the scales.

Healthful carbohydrates include fruits, potatoes, grains, beans, and rice. If you study the U.S. Department of Agriculture's recommended food pyramid (see page 102), you'll see the base of the pyramid is given over to carbohydrates. They hold up the rest of a healthful diet!

Whatever your chosen master diet plan that targets weight-loss and a healthy life, give carbohydrates a major role. You may find that they become your preferred foods.

*Eliminate Extras*
*Sugar*

Refined sugar is suspected of contributing to everything from arthritis to impotence. Some nutritionists claim that refined sugar is the cause of hypoglycemia, a condition that may afflict as many as twenty million Americans. (Hypoglycemia, or low blood sugar, can cause dizziness, irritability, anxiety, insomnia, depression, loss of sex drive, and even nervous breakdowns.) And it's not just the body that succumbs to sugar. For years, dentists have blamed sticky cereals, chewy candy, and syrupy soft drinks as the major cavity-causing culprits.

Why, then, knowing what we know, do we continue to eat more and more refined sugar each year? "Our tastes are conditioned from the day we're born," explains Dr. Eleanor Williams, author and nutrition professor at Buffalo State University. "Sugar is a hidden additive in baby food, vegetables, processed meats, and bread and predisposes us to crave even more highly sweetened foods." Many foods you wouldn't expect to have a high sugar content: hot dogs, canned vegetables, peanut butter, and catsup, just to name a few. Sugar is a cheap filler which food processors use to take up space in food. So much of our sugar intake comes from processed foods, we don't know how much we're really getting.

When we overweight people work to lose weight or to maintain a natural weight, we certainly don't expect to be sabotaged by a can of tomatoes. The simple key to identifying hidden sugar is to read food labels. Federal regulations require that ingredients be listed by grams and in order of quantity. If the product you're buying has sugar as the second or third ingredient, it's got too much sugar for your diet. And watch out for sugar in other forms, such as sucrose, fructose, rice syrup, and corn syrup.

Another drawback to a high-sugar diet is mood disorders. "Sugar in candy and pastries did crazy things to me," admitted one dieter to her group. "About a half hour after consuming a lot of it, I'd get dizzy and very drowsy. Sometimes I would go to bed, sleep two or three hours, and wake up feeling hungover. My mood was awful. I was easily agitated and bad-tempered over everything."

Not every overeater has this reaction to consuming too much sugar. Some of us just get fat. But if sugar seems to cause you physical and mood changes in addition to gaining weight, inform your doctor. Dieters who have had negative reactions to refined sugar may decide to live without it. Many people who eliminate white sugar from their diets say it is surprisingly simple to do. After about seventy-six hours, the craving for sweets leaves and does not return unless it is fueled again with more sugar.

*Salt*

The warning is out: Too much salt can endanger your health. Using far more salt than your body requires can lead to high blood pressure and kidney disease.

Eliminate salt from your cooking, or if you must use it, add a little at the end of the cooking process so the salt taste comes first to the palate and quickly satisfies. Unless you are cooking with fresh ingredients, the manufacturer may have already salted the product during processing. Since almost all foods, even drinking water, contain some sodium, taste before you salt.

Why do we need to watch our salt intake more carefully than thin people? Because fluid retention is one of the consequences of extra salt. The body must maintain a critical balance of salt and water, but the sodium in salt absorbs water, causing us to drink more and show a weight gain. We don't need that.

We may have spicy appetites, liking food on the overseasoned side, but we can train our taste buds to respond to less salty food, which may even help us lose weight. Better health and more weight loss—that's not a bad payoff for using a lighter hand on the salt shaker.

*Caffeine*

Studies have shown that overweight people tend to consume too much caffeine—in the form of coffee, tea, or cola. One reason for such excessive consumption is that caffeine creates a craving. Whenever caffeine "addicts" try to stop, they suffer withdrawal-like symptoms, including depression, nervousness, and a decrease in alertness.

Other symptoms, such as fatigue, nervousness, and headaches, often accompany heavy coffee or cola drinking. If you feel that caffeine is a problem, cut down or consult your doctor.

How much caffeine is okay? Your intake must be based on your reaction to caffeine. Tune in to your body. It will tell you if you are getting too much caffeine.

Excess caffeine, like too much food, is a crutch we sometimes use to prop up our personalities. But no matter how firmly rooted in our need for a crutch, we can replace it when we realize that our new healthy life will give us all the energy and mental sharpness we need.

*Include Essentials*
*Water*

Most of us look for a cold drink many times a day. Too often, we reach for sodas and iced teas that have too much sugar and caffeine. Carbonated diet sodas often are too gaseous for constant use. Fruit juices have too many concentrated sugar calories to be used as hourly thirst quenchers. Fortunately, we can satisfy our thirst by consuming the perfect beverage: water.

Plenty of plain water—eight to ten eight-ounce glasses a day—in addition to quenching our thirst without adding an ounce of weight, cleanses and purifies our bodies, improving our general health.

To encourage yourself to drink more water, try putting an insulated water jug or cooler in your refrigerator—one with a spigot to make it handier to use. For a real treat, try filling it with bottled spring water, which often tastes better than tap water. Add a slice of lemon or lime for a fresh taste.

During the hot summer months, it's not unusual to consume sixty-four ounces of liquid a day or twice that amount if you are exercising. If all your liquids contained calories, hot-weather dieting would be more difficult than necessary.

Again, switching to water is a matter of mind-set and determination to get as close as you can to maximum health.

### Vitamins

To take vitamins or not is a question many dieters ask. Do you really need them? If you eat a varied diet and are in good health, you are probably getting enough vitamins. Sometimes when we are on weight-losing diets, our doctors will suggest a multivitamin just to be on the safe side. There's nothing dangerous about a moderate supplement approved by your doctor.

But be careful. Excesses of some vitamins can be toxic, especially of vitamins A and D.

And although vitamin C has many claims made for it—from curing the common cold to protecting against cancers caused by chemical pollution—too much vitamin C can destroy vitamin B-12, with anemia the possible consequence. If you have chosen a primarily starch-based diet instead of meat and dairy, you may want to take a B-12 supplement to guard against a deficiency.

Most of our vitamin needs are met through a healthy diet. We can control our vitamin intake through our food choices. For example, vitamins A, C, and E are antioxidants—substances that protect our cells from damage and thus may reduce our risk of cancer, heart and lung disease, and even cataracts. We can easily add antioxidants to our diets naturally by eating fruits and vegetables, especially broccoli, cantaloupe, pink grapefruit, collard greens, kale, mangoes, spinach, winter squash, and sweet potatoes.

When it comes to vitamins, we dieters need to heed a familiar refrain: everything in moderation. It turns out that most of us can get all the vitamins we need naturally, especially if we're eating nutrient-rich foods, which, for us, is a happier possibility than swallowing pills.

But remember that different people have different nutritional needs. Check with your doctor or nutritionist about yours—don't rely on the vitamin advice of friends or neighbors.

*Minerals*

A balanced supply of minerals is also crucial for your health—they are "the basic spark plugs in the chemistry of life." However, you only need them in minute amounts.

The list of trace minerals you need for biochemical and physiological health reads like a geology student's final exam: fluorine, chromium, manganese, iron, cobalt, copper, zinc, molybdenum, and iodine. There are dozens of other elements that occur in concentrations too small to measure, which work in thousands of intricate ways. Deficiencies, while rare in an age that supplies fresh fruits and vegetables year-round, can cause serious health problems. For example, lack of iodine causes goiter. Lack of fluorine causes weak bones and poor teeth. And if you don't get enough iron, you become anemic.

The right proportion *between* minerals seems to be one key to good health for dieters. For example, take the three elements cadmium, zinc, and copper. Too much copper in proportion to zinc may cause high blood cholesterol. Too much cadmium may result from eating highly refined foods. Too much zinc can result from eating a diet too high in fats. Excessive mineral supplements, calcium for example, could inhibit iron absorption.

The solution to all these potential problems is this: except during certain times (such as pregnancy), mineral supplements are probably not necessary *if you eat a healthful, balanced diet.*

*Fiber*

Most Americans eat 12 to 15 grams of dietary fiber a day, only half the 25 grams of soluble and insoluble fiber the U.S. Department of Agriculture recommends. Where can we get all that fiber?

It actually adds up quickly in a healthy, whole foods diet. A slice of whole-wheat bread contains 2 grams; a cup of brown rice, 3 grams; a cup of bran cereal, 9 grams; one-half cup prunes, 7 grams; one cup blackberries, 8.9 grams; one ear of corn, 8 grams; and one orange, 5 grams. The ideal diet contains a combination of soluble and insoluble fibers.

Soluble fiber, which lowers cholesterol, is found in oat bran, fruits, vegetables, beans, lentils, and peas.

Insoluble fiber, which lowers cholesterol and reduces the incidence of colon cancer, is found in wheat bran, fruits, vegetables, and whole grains such as corn, rye, barley, and brown rice. A mix of both fibers is ideal in our daily diet, and contributes to a healthier lifestyle.

Increase your intake of high-fiber foods gradually. Rapid changes may overstimulate your digestive system and provoke gastrointestinal distress. But do eat more fiber. Not only will you promote your good health, but you'll be adding more filling foods to your diet, which will make it easier to stick with your master eating plan.

## Exercise—It's Your Time to Play

The role that regular physical exercise plays in the loss and management of weight is something that most of us talk about, but all too few of us ever do anything about. And yet the reality is that in any program of *fat* control, exercise (which is simply the expenditure of stored fat energy) is extremely important. Think of what farmers do when they want to fatten cattle. They restrict their activity by confining them in small areas, *where the animals can get no exercise.* If you want to deliberately fatten yourself, refrain from most exercise. If you want to unfatten yourself, do the opposite.

But losing fat isn't the only way your body will benefit from exercise. Here's what happens when you exercise: living cells constantly metabolize. Oxygen and nutrients move in and waste moves out. The number of red blood cells increases, clotting time is lowered, and blood delivers more oxygen to all the body cells. The vitality of every single cell depends upon nutrition and *activity.*

The sedentary nature of your way of living has upset the energy equation of your life. Your job is to set it right again. Couple a healthy diet with regular exercise, and you will soon have your body functioning the way it was meant to.

You'll have to unlearn some old habits. Overweight people are remarkably adept at accomplishing physical tasks with the least amount of effort. That's the paradox of energy—if you store it, you lose it; if you spend it, you have it. While it may pay off in dollars to conserve electric and gas energy, it does not pay off to conserve your own energy.

Exercise is an obvious way to use up energy stored as extra fat on your body. The difference between walking and driving three miles to work is approximately an eighteen-pound-per-year weight loss. And that is without changing your diet.

Look at your body as more than an eating machine. In simplest terms, your body is a chemical furnace that burns food to produce energy. But what happens to the energy once it's produced is up to you. It can be stored in fat cells, or it can be expended in activity.

*Overweight and underactive* in today's society seem to go hand in hand. Our ancestors walked and worked from sunup to sundown. They didn't worry about proper exercise. It was built into their lives. That's not true today.

Whether you're an executive, a mother, or an astronaut you're smart to exercise. Keep in mind that if you're more than 20 percent overweight or have any medical condition, your doctor needs to okay your exercise program.

In addition, anyone over thirty years old embarking on an exercise program ought to have a thorough examination first. And, if you're over forty years old, you should be checked for heart disease.

If you follow a balanced exercise program, you'll improve your body's vital organs and limbs, build up the efficiency of your heart and lungs, add to your muscular strength and endurance, and improve your balance, flexibility, and agility. And while you're perspiring, that fat will be melting away so that you'll be firm and fit.

In addition, exercise before a meal has been found to dull the appetite, thereby causing you to eat less. And not only will you consume fewer calories, but you'll also burn up to twice as many calories following vigorous exercise as you do normally.

As little as thirty minutes of exercise every day can take off as much as twenty-six pounds a year if you keep your calorie count the same. And it's *regular exercise,* rather than exercise intensity, that is more important. Only twenty minutes of exercise three times a week can be beneficial for losing weight and improving general health. For an idea of how many calories you burn through exercise, consult the chart below.

Yes, you can lose weight without exercise, but you'll be missing a marvelous body experience. After a few sessions, you are going to feel more limber and more alive. Besides, those new clothes will look better on a toned body.

Number of calories burned per minute for 120-pound adult. Add 5 percent more calories for each additional 10-pound increment.

| *Activity* | *Calories Burned* |
| --- | --- |
| Aerobic dance | 6.2 |
| Basketball | 4.3 |
| Bicycling (12 mph) | 9.0 |
| Canoeing (4 mph) | 5.7 |
| Football | 4.3 |
| Gymnastics | 4.4 |
| Hiking | 4.3 |

| *Activity* | *Calories Burned* |
| --- | --- |
| Jogging (5.5 mph) | 9.2 |
| Skating | 5.0 |
| Skiing (cross-country) | 9.9 |
| Soccer | 7.7 |
| Softball | 4.0 |
| Swimming | 8.8 |
| Tennis (doubles) | 4.0 |
| Tennis (singles) | 6.0 |
| Volleyball | 5.0 |
| Walking (2 mph) | 3.0 |
| Walking (4.5 mph) | 5.5 |
| Weight training | 6.7 |

*What Exercise Is Right for You?*

There are four categories of exercise—isometrics, isotonics, anaerobics, and aerobics. Each one fills a specific physical need.

*Isometrics.* Isometric exercise promotes muscular strength and bulk through contractions. This is accomplished by pushing or pulling against an immovable object, such as a door frame, or by pitting one group of muscles against another.

*Isotonics.* These exercises are a new-fangled name for the old-fashioned toe touches, push-ups, and sit-ups that your high school gym teacher called calisthenics. They serve mainly to limber up or to condition the body. Not-too-active sports such as shuffleboard and pitching horseshoes are also isotonic exercises.

*Anaerobics.* A fifty-yard dash, weight lifting, and racquetball are good examples of this exercise, which builds endurance and stamina.

*Aerobics.* This is the fat burner. It increases heart and respiratory action for a sustained period of time.

Running, cross-country skiing, rowing, jumping rope, cycling, and swimming all fall into this category of exercise.

Exercise in any form burns calories, but you have another mission—total body fitness. Developing a balanced exercise program that uses some parts of several of these exercise disciplines will help your body retain protein and minerals, increase oxygen in red blood cells, promote digestion, boost heart efficiency, increase stamina and tone muscles.

To be this effective, your exercise program should include an aerobic workout of enough intensity to stimulate heart-lung function, and, most important, it should be *regular*. Walking, bicycling, swimming, rope-skipping, or even following a workout video in the privacy of your bedroom will burn up calories and make you feel better. And the greater the variety of exercise, the better. Athletes call it cross-training. Which exercises should you try? All of them. Open your mind to every sport or exercise that catches your fancy. Versatility is the spice of exercise.

You've felt mentally and physically low for long enough. With a little exercise, you will gain more energy than you expend. You can use that extra energy to get more out of living.

Remember to build in safeguards so that you will stick to your exercise plan. Don't set up a program that will consume too much of your time at first. You can always expand your program later. It's better to exercise twenty minutes a day every day than in sporadic spurts of heavy exercise on the weekend. The physical benefits of occasional exercise reverse themselves within a matter of days.

To get the most out of exercise and to stay with it, you need to enjoy yourself. If it's a bore or a chore, you may give up too soon. Try exercises you enjoy or that you think you'll enjoy. If you're comfortable doing so, exercise with a pal or group—doing it alone may be hard at first. A friend may provide the encouragement you need to keep going. As with many new experiences, the first few days are the most difficult. After that, pride and just plain feeling better will help make exercising easier than you ever thought it would be.

If you tend to be one of those who resists a formal exercise program, you can sneak in a great deal of exercise without feeling it—except in a trimmer body:

1. When you go shopping at the mall or supermarket, park as far back in the parking lot as is safe and walk to the store.

2. Don't take elevators when you can climb stairs.

3. Instead of hiring yard or housework done, do it yourself, and put muscle into it.

4. Bicycle or walk short distances for shopping or visiting.

These are only a few of the ways you can change your habits to use food energy. You can probably think of others.

### The Benefits of Basic Exercises

When examining workout possibilities, it's important to note that some have very specific benefits for us.

#### Swimming

No exercise is easier than swimming if you're overweight. You may not be able to jog, walk, or cycle on a par with more physically fit people, but the buoyancy of water is a great equalizer. You'll be able to swim as well as anyone.

Once in the water, relax, keep your legs straight and "grip" the water. Swimming pros suggest you think of the water as gelatin—grab hold of it and push off with your body. Work on endurance by using a smooth stroke that will carry you some distance. Don't just float in the water. You'll get no more exercise than in your bathtub.

*Running*

Does running for exercise sound impossible? Do you believe overweight people can't run? If you answer yes, you're wrong. Not only is it possible, but it can lead to beautiful results.

Running is best eased into with a walk-jog-run program as outlined by physical fitness expert Joe Henderson.

Henderson suggests a two-month walking program, with jogging starting in the third month. Jogs can vary from one minute to five minutes, with 90 percent of them in the two-to-four-minute range.

After three months, you can progress to running. Most people in Henderson's program run twenty minutes.

Another way to approach running, says Dr. Ralph S. Paffenbarger Jr. of the University of California, is to start out walking until you get to the point where you can walk three and a half to four miles in an hour— that's a pretty fast clip. It will take a few weeks to build up to this rate, so have patience.

Next, walk for five minutes, followed by a five-minute jog, until you can build up to a thirty-minute jog with a five minute warm-up and cool-down at least three times a week. "But watch for any signs of chest pain or joint pain," warns Dr. Paffenbarger, "and stop immediately if they appear."

When you and your doctor agree you are ready to begin the running stage of your exercise buildup, remember to take it easy. Run at a gentle pace. To evaluate your pace, take the "talk test." If you can't talk in complete sentences without gasping, slow down. On the other hand, if you're not breathing harder than normal, work harder.

*Weight Lifting*

Lifting weights has always been a favorite way for men to turn flesh into muscle, but it's also beneficial for women. Female hormones just don't allow muscles to mass as they do on men, so women can use weights to tone and firm their bodies.

Weight lifting is also a good way to build strength and stamina for either gender. Weight lifters find they begin to improve in other areas of exercise. Their aerobic performance increases and they have energy to spare.

Many dieters find weight lifting more challenging and satisfying than plain exercising because they can see progress in the increased poundage they lift. That alone keeps a person interested, and maintaining interest is what many people find the hardest part of any exercise routine.

Remember to warm up before any exercise. Cold muscles burn sugar; warm muscles burn fat, and you're on a fat-burning trip. Cool down after vigorous exercise to allow your heart to gradually reach its normal rate.

There's no argument that exercise is important to weight loss and good body tone. Any way you do it, with weights or without, you're bound to get a lift.

*Home-Exercise Machines*

Although you don't need expensive equipment to get good exercise, you may want to own a machine so you can work out with maximum convenience and privacy.

A number of machines on the market combine a good aerobic workout with strength training. Most have digital readouts so that you can keep track of elapsed time, number of repetitions, and calories expended. A fifty-minute machine workout can burn as many as 1,000 calories of fat and work every major muscle group. Your arms, legs, shoulders, and back all work together, giving you the feeling of being a powerful person. As a bonus, many of these machines are low-impact, so they take it easy on your joints and bones.

Since exercise machines can cost from $100 to $700 or more, try several types of machines before you buy, and purchase an instructional video for your machine if one is available. It will help you keep the right pace and show you the correct way to use the equipment so that you won't injure yourself. Be willing to invest in your healthy new life. You're worth it.

## The Benefits of Positive Doing

When we overeaters think about eating, we tend to dwell on the "kick" we got out of certain foods, the pleasure, the escape from boredom, the release from fear or anger, and the companionship of eating with others—especially when they are overeating.

What we don't think about is the physical unpleasantness: bloating, gas, nausea; or the emotional unpleasantness: the remorse, the waste of precious time, and the facing of another day fatter than we were before.

To be losing weight or to be maintaining a natural weight is to get a real "kick" out of life. Overeating may have given us a temporary sense of exhilaration, but it didn't last. It was too soon followed by incredible guilt, anguish, and utter desolation. Sometimes, on the morning after, we were inconsolable in our grief—grief for our bodies, grief for our shredded feelings, and a special grief over what might be if only we could get control of our eating.

In truth, self-control is the real kick for people like

us. Losing weight is the real kick. Living without constant self-recrimination is the real kick.

Day after day you are eating for health and are growing as a person. The initial flames of your exciting new life will someday die down to a mellow glow. But this is maturing that can bring you real comfort as you put one good day after another behind you. Healthful, growth-oriented days are the most richly rewarding days we former overeaters can spend. But such success requires self-understanding, time, and careful handling.

Give it to yourself.

## A Note from the Author about Her Personal Health Plan

Just like many of you, I have a long history of losing weight, regaining it, losing it, and regaining it again.

I went on my first weight-losing diet when I was twelve. My mother took me to the doctor after she found me crying because other children wouldn't allow me to play with them. The family doctor found nothing wrong with me except that I needed to lose thirty pounds. He handed my mother a diet sheet of recommended foods and serving amounts. It was my first diet and I did lose weight, but two years later I was back in the doctor's office, this time forty pounds overweight. He handed out the same diet sheet. "But I've already tried this diet," I said. "Don't you have something better?" "Just eat less," he replied. "There's nothing more I can do for you."

I was on my own, and over the next twenty years I yo-yoed between thin, plump, fat, and "morbidly obese" (in medical terms), gaining hundreds of pounds, trying every popular diet regimen, pills, even bypass surgery (later reversed), until I topped out at 272 pounds. At last I lost over 100 pounds and have kept that fat off for more than twenty years. My personal eating plan for that weight loss and maintenance was the basic four food groups plan, since replaced with the U.S. Department of Agriculture's food pyramid, shown on page 102.

*My Eating Plan*

Originally my diet was primarily protein-centered: meat and cheese, with large salads and some fruit, but almost no starches. I weighed portions and counted calories. This diet worked very well for a long time, except for one problem—after forming new and positive attitudes toward food and myself, I still spent considerable energy every day fighting real hunger; yet I could not increase my caloric intake without gaining weight, even with exercise.

This is the way it has to be, I thought, and I determined to make it work, whatever it took.

A few years ago, I discovered a satisfying new way of eating while trying to help my husband change his eating habits after heart surgery. At first, I was reluctant to study the heart dietary guidelines and attend special cooking classes to learn to cook without added oil. After all, who knew more about diets than I did?

But I relented, and to my surprise I soon learned that there is a lot more to diet and nutrition than weight loss and maintenance. I was exposed to the concept of maximum health and the very low-fat (less than 10 percent of daily calories), starch-centered diet. The more I read and attended seminars by two of the gurus of this way of eating, internist Dr. John McDougall and heart specialist Dr. Dean Ornish, the more I wondered if such a diet could be for me. My husband was dealing with a potentially fatal disease; I was convinced it would be good for him.

The diet was simple. I just lopped off the top of the U.S.D.A. food pyramid, as the Physicians Committee for Responsible Medicine (a vegetarian advocacy group) has done here.

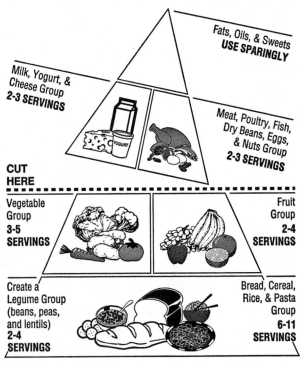

Source: U.S. Department of Agriculture

First to go was all added fat during cooking, then meat and eggs, which were the easiest for me. Dairy products, however, were much harder. I had used milk as a beverage and eaten cheese daily all of my life. At first, I went to the low-fat varieties, but they still contained more fat than I wanted. It took several months before I'd totally eliminated dairy products from my eating plan.

"So what is there left to eat?" my friends ask, some truly concerned that I must be starving. "Every good plant under the sun," is my answer. After several years, I remain honestly astounded at the variety of delicious foods I can eat: rice, corn, legumes, potatoes, whole grains, homemade pasta, fresh vegetables, and fruits. And as a bonus, cooking has become an exciting and creative activity once again.

On my new low-fat, starch-centered diet, I started to lose weight again, slowly and steadily, about two pounds a month, until I'd lost an additional twenty pounds. (Others on similar programs report losses from six to fifteen pounds per month.)

And I am measurably healthier. All my medical tests are normal or better. My cholesterol dropped to 150.

Even the federal government has assured Americans that vegetarian diets are consistent with the dietary guidelines as long as the variety and amounts of foods consumed are adequate.

My way of eating is one that I came to after half a life-time of experimentation. It's not for everyone; it takes more time to buy and prepare fresh, whole foods, and you need to know more about nutrition than the average dieter. It's very important to consult your physician about your personal nutritional needs. I consulted several doctors and dietitians, and I constantly fine-tuned my diet according to the latest nutritional information.

I am not qualified to make medical claims, and I'm not doing so here. I can only tell you what happened to me: my migraine headaches ceased, my joint pain disappeared, my upset stomachs are a memory.

But the *best* result of my new diet came early and stayed late. I no longer feel hunger between meals. I am now giving my body what it has always wanted—the healthiest possible food.

## *My Exercise Plan*

For much of my life, I was extremely sedentary. The mere thought of physical exercise conjured up the extreme embarrassment of high school gym class. But when I lost one hundred pounds, I wanted to get in shape as well. I wanted to have a firm, toned body and a great deal more energy. *I wanted to be fit.*

But the discipline eluded me. Soon my hall closet and garage were littered with next-to-new exercise equipment and clothing left over from failed attempts to force myself to be more active.

By the time my optometrist mentioned that bifocals loomed on my horizon, I was ready to try again. And this time I determined not to be an exercise flop. Remembering that games were the one thing I'd liked about gym, I decided to find a fun game to play that would give me a good workout.

I chose tennis, since there were tennis courts near my house. It was a good choice since it prevented my using the old "it takes too much time to get there" excuse. I also signed and posted a typed contract with myself so that I wouldn't "forget" or "be too busy." In the contract, I agreed to take lessons and play tennis three times a week for two months. By the end of the two months, I liked tennis (and winning) so much that I didn't want to stop; I also liked my newfound energy and stamina.

But the result that really pressed my exercise button was body contour. I looked better in my clothes and out of them. That hooked me on exercise. Over the years, I've added other exercises, targeting maximum health. I lift weights for strength and increased bone density; I walk, hike, and bicycle. I enjoy being in the open air, and the diversity keeps me from ever becoming bored.

Back in the beginning of my exercise odyssey, it wasn't always easy for me to maintain a physically active life but as benefit piled on top of benefit—weight loss, flexibility, body sculpting, fat melt-down, stronger bones, and a wonderful sense of well-being—exercise became an essential part of my life. Now I manage to squeeze it in even on the busiest days. It's my turn to play.

Curing your weight problem with a healthy food and exercise plan will not only make you feel your best; it will make you look your best too. Thin and healthy is the payoff. But before attaining this reward, you must carefully set the stage for success.

# CHAPTER 5

# Positive Living

## Maintaining Your New Lifestyle

*A*nn Richards, former Governor of Texas, once pointed out that, while Fred Astaire is often extravagantly praised, "Ginger Rogers did everything that Fred Astaire did. She just did it backwards and in high heels." If you feel your life has been one long backwards dance, it's time *you* took the lead and danced in your own direction. That's what *The Thin Books* is all about: helping you take the initiative to make good things happen.

By this time you've surely learned that you're not "incurably fat." There's no such disease. You have choices, and you are capable of making them. Despite every obstacle you've faced, you have at last begun to value yourself, to trust yourself, to give yourself the chance you need to lead a thin, healthy, active life—the life you've always wanted.

Why, then, deep down, are you still a little afraid? "Can I really stick to it this time?" That's the question we all ask ourselves. With our diet history, fear of failing is common, especially after we've experienced some benefits and would like to experience even more. What you need is answers.

This chapter is all about sticking to it, dealing with

cravings and the stress that can lead to relapse, and learning techniques that will make you strong. You'll be able to keep what you've achieved and prepare to go even further.

Eighty percent of life, as actor/director Woody Allen says, is showing up. And you've done just that as you've made a passage through these pages. You are in the midst of custom-tailoring a way of living that matches your deepest desire. You have positive new responses to destructive thoughts and feelings that formerly led in only one direction—feeding them. Daily, even hourly, you are facing your anger, guilt, or frustration and choosing not to use extra food to stuff those feelings back down inside. Observing yourself honestly is an integral part of your positive new attitude. *You've shown up for your own life.*

Having an upbeat attitude is an important part of being a healthy person—studies repeatedly show that it's one of the predictors of longevity. And the best way to get and keep a positive outlook is to take an active role in managing your own health. Victims wait for the sky to fall; achievers take control.

A prime example is a man named Noel Johnson who by his late sixties was so obese that it was all he could do to lift his hand to his mouth. His doctor told him his heart would give out in six months. Noel decided he didn't have much to lose, so he started a diet—and walking.

Sure enough, he died—at age ninety-five, after he set age records for a quarter century running marathons and had his picture on a Wheaties box, at age seventy-seven, as an exemplar of fitness.

It's not too late for you, either. Now is the time to take a long look at what you'd like to confront and change in your life. Are there things holding you back—at work or at home? Don't give up because of these barriers, but view them as challenges and meet them head on. Decide to tackle one problem today, and take a first step in your own marathon. Tomorrow, confront another nagging problem. The more you create a sense of self-control, the more you will think, "Hey, I'm doing a lot for myself." Can you imagine how good that will make you feel?

Putting your goals in writing is a great way to continue this positive upward trend. What's the next thing you want to do for your body? "I want to be thin," is not specific enough. "I want to lose ten pounds in six weeks," will work better. Take a look at your fitness goals, and write down how far you want to walk, jog, or bike in one month. Remember when you write it down, you commit to it.

Now that you're in charge, you're on the way to being your own personal success story. Say yes to that.

## Sticking to It

Most of us are grateful for our new way of life. To be free of the compulsion to overeat, to be healthy in body and spirit—these mean a great deal to us. A life well-lived is worth more than any fortune imaginable. And that is exactly what you are aiming for—a healthy, active life lived to the utmost.

At this point, it might be interesting to remember just how you got to be worth so much. You took four simple yet giant steps forward. First, you admitted you had a problem with food; second, you believed you could do something about it; third, you expressed a desire to change; and fourth, you became willing to work for that change.

That's it. Four simple steps led you onto a new life

path. But your work isn't done. Healthy eating and continued inner growth is a big job, one that will last your lifetime. You must work on it every day.

Your weight-losing experience has definitely taught you to pay attention to *what, when, and how much you eat; your real hunger; and your need for physical activity.* This careful attention will also help you as you switch from a weight-loss plan to a weight-maintenance plan.

In some ways, even after you move into maintenance, your lifestyle will need little change. As you adjust your intake to end weight loss and keep your weight stable, you'll want to do the following:

1. Keep a close weight check as you increase calories. Weigh yourself regularly, and whenever your scale shows two or three pounds over your target weight, return to your weight-losing eating plan. Set your upper limit based on your own history. You'll know when it's time to cut back.

2. Eat regular meals. High-calorie snacking is never for the "formerly fat."

3. Start from your weight-losing plan, slowly adding higher calorie foods to your diet, *one food at a time.* Watch the scale to see how your body responds to each addition before adding more.

4. Eat a healthy diet based on sound nutritional information.

5. Exercise several times a week.

To keep extra pounds from creeping back on a receptive body requires courage. Courage is the ability to survive defeat, disappointment, and loss without looking for that old destructive "drug"—food.

Weight maintenance also requires a good memory. You must never forget how you felt when your dress or pant size was so large you could only buy from a specialty store. You must never forget that a short walk was exhausting, a longer walk, impossible. Nor must you forget how your loved ones worried about your health.

You have the courage and the determination to maintain your weight loss. And you certainly have the memory. But outside factors will inevitably challenge your healthier lifestyle and threaten your weight maintenance. It's important to recognize these factors and find ways to deal with them.

*Priorities—What Comes First*

A dieter was heard to comment after stepping away from her weekly weigh-in: "It's no wonder I haven't lost any weight. I've been trying to sell my home, take care of three teenagers, keep up my golf lessons, and start a computer course."

That's not an empty excuse. It's a wonder she could stick to any eating plan, trying to do so many things at once. What comes first in every dieter's life? We need to eliminate the confusion, hurry, and anxiety that doing too much creates. If there is one time in your life when you should set priorities, it's now, when you are trying to cope with your food problem.

Set your priorities and place *eating to live,* instead of *living to eat,* at the head of your list. Concentrate on this one thing. You have set a goal for healthy weight loss. Now examine what you are doing to reach that goal. Ask yourself the following questions:

1. What am I doing to accomplish the results I want? Am I in charge or am I relying on others, such as a doctor or a weight-loss pill?

2. In the light of the self-knowledge I've gained, is my original goal realistic? Sometimes in the first flush of determination, we set a goal that is impossible, then become frustrated and give up. Why not revise your goal before you get to the giving-up stage?

3. What has my achievement so far taught me about what I can expect of myself in the future? Our accomplishments teach us what we need to know for future goal-setting if we really assess them honestly.

Remember that moving toward your goal is a journey. You will run into both obstacles and opportunities. This is no small or short journey, so be patient and stay on track.

Many of us tend to forget that a "diet," in the sense that we overeaters use the term, is not a plan of eating for a few days, weeks, or even months. The word *diet* comes from the Latin *diaeta* and the Greek *diaita,* both meaning "way of life." We are entering into a permanent new way of life.

Every dieter wonders, "How long will it take me to lose my weight?" It's a reasonable question. We wouldn't be trying so hard if we weren't anxious to start a new life in a new body. Although it may have taken years to gain our excess weight, we would like to have it disappear overnight.

There's nothing wrong with a little impatience. It helps give us our drive and pushes us to get jobs done. But too much impatience can push you to the point of despair: "I've been on this diet a whole week and only lost three pounds. I quit!"

Impatience is especially hurtful to people trying to *maintain* healthy eating programs. It is all too easy to slip from impatience into despair, and then trade despair for a numbing food binge.

The best way to develop patience is to learn to be realistic about the rhythms of living. You can seldom write a timetable for your life and expect everything and everybody to fall into line. It's far better to live a day at a time. Excitement can keep you going in the beginning of your new regimen, but what's most important is the everyday march toward your weight goal—not how long it takes.

Change, especially the change of lifelong eating habits, is a slow process. It takes a whole lifetime. Many of us used to think that once we lost our weight, we would be thin forever and nothing we ate would ever make us fat again. Unfortunately, there is no never-never land where we can eat whatever and whenever we want. We will always have to practice healthy eating habits.

If you honestly follow a new health program, your excess weight will come off. We may not always lose as fast as we want, but our bodies lose as fast as they should. Learn to respect your body's time tables.

Difficult as it is to cultivate patience, it's equally tough to resist the tempting promises of quick fixes. Like the old-time medicine man selling snake oil cures, an ever-increasing number of diet gadgets promise instant relief from fat. The long list includes pills, thigh creams, and "amazing" skin patches.

We overweight people cannot rely on gadgets to help us lose weight. If you must lean on something, lean on yourself. Actively take the initiative. You alone determine your destiny through your own efforts. Do you want to lose weight? Then establish a master plan for eating and exercising to do it. Do you want to change your destructive emotional patterns? Then establish a positive master plan for inner growth.

Success in changing your lifestyle results when you combine adaptability with activity. If you are not losing weight on your present eating plan, get another. It's good enough for you only if it works.

*Measuring Progress*

As if slow change wasn't difficult enough, we are also surrounded by constant reminders of how we look and what we weigh. These readily available measuring devices—scales and mirrors—are important tools, but they often add to our sense of urgency.

More than four million new scales are sold every year. That means a lot of us follow the little needle from pound to pound. The great debate isn't whether it's a good idea to keep track of your weight, but how often you should do it.

Doctors generally insist on weighing patients at the beginning of each visit. Most doctors' offices are equipped with giant digital scales that can be absolutely overwhelming in their accuracy—especially if you haven't lost weight since your last office call. Even home scales, while weighing lighter as a rule, are just as menacing to some dieters. But they can become a dieter's best friend, if used regularly.

How often should you weigh yourself? Most diet clubs have rules about weighing. Some weight-loss groups prefer their members not hop on the scale between weekly class weigh-ins. On the other hand, some behavior therapy groups insist on daily weighing with corresponding weight charts, although they discourage compulsive weighing at all times of the day or night.

Some groups suggest weighing only once a month to prevent members from becoming too easily discouraged at a slow weight loss or overly excited by a quick one. Diets, they say, have been broken for either of these two reasons.

Most dieters find a comfortable weighing plan somewhere in between, based on their doctor's wishes, the rules of their diet group, and their own preferences. The trick is not to give too much power to your scale. Some people allow a drop in pounds to trigger increased eating. If you're honest with yourself, you'll use the scales to determine only how much weight you're losing, not how much more food you can eat.

On the other hand, your bathroom scale can be one of the greatest motivators to keep you going. Stepping on the scale and finding you've broken another "pound barrier" is a great thrill. Since we have an emotional response to our body weight, dropping below the weight we were last year at this time, or when the baby was born, or when we were married can give us a special motivation to continue dieting.

The best way to integrate your scale into your new, thin life is to switch it to the role of friendly monitor. This will be its lifelong job. When your scale shows a weight gain of two to three pounds, it will immediately trigger your new behavior—a return to your weight-loss program until the extra weight is gone. Remember what you used to say? "It's probably just that time of month," or, "I'll cut back next Monday"? That old system of postponement didn't work, and before you knew it, you were ten or twenty pounds overweight again, feeling hopeless and helpless.

When it comes time to say good-bye to your old motivator, just turn around and say hello to your friendly monitor—the best watchdog your new body will ever know.

Learn to use other motivators to prove your progress. You have another real friend in your measuring tape. When you're losing weight, you're not just losing pounds, but inches—lots and lots of inches. "I couldn't believe it," said one woman who reached her target weight, "but when I added all my lost inches together, they totaled 137, more than *twice* my own height."

You'll be cheating yourself out of some real fun and

fulfillment if you don't measure yourself occasionally. Once a week, measure your waistline, bust, abdomen, hips, upper thighs, calves, ankles, upper and lower arms. Make a chart and keep a weekly record. Although the scale sometimes gets stuck for a discouraging time, your measurements may continue to go down.

Be aware that overweight people seem to lose first what they need to lose least, and lose last what they need to lose most. Your face, bust, and waist may be normal in size long before your hips catch up. Don't despair—they will pare down eventually, if you stick with your diet and exercise regimen long enough.

## What Keeps Getting You Down?

The toughest part of any diet comes when we see the progress we've worked so hard to achieve slipping away. Beware of falling into the old "What's the use of trying?" attitude.

When we get on the scales to discover we've gained weight, that's tough, but it's not final. *There is real hope for you.* You can get back on track today and for all the days of your life.

Try to determine what keeps getting you down? Often, it's guilt, frustration, and other negative feelings that underlie depression. That's why, when you get down, you give up. And then you keep on feeling worse and worse.

The key is to *keep sticking to your plan.* Do what you have to do, whether it's easy or not. You'll like your healthy eating results well enough—the new body, the new positive mental attitude. Sometimes we sit around waiting for inspiration to strike us. It rarely does. Inspiration comes from *doing* what we have to do, not *thinking* about it. *Action* is your magic word.

Of course, this is all much easier said than done. How

do you keep optimistic when you feel terrible about a few pounds that have crept back on? How do you stick to your diet when someone has broken your heart and all you want to do is curl up with a carton of chocolate-chip-cookie-dough ice cream?

There are tools that can help you cope and ways to work through the emotions that tempt you to return to overeating. You are not alone. Help is at hand, and there are more coping options than Haägen Dazs flavors. And you are strong enough to choose the right path. Believe it.

*Concentration—Focus on It*

Concentration is a tool you'll need in order to stay on your healthy new plan. Eastern philosophers call concentration the master art, because all other arts depend on it. How do you develop your power of concentration? Through practice, of course, just like any art.

Concentration, simply stated, is paying full attention to what is happening at the moment. When you concentrate, you are able to experience losing weight more fully.

During a diet group meeting, a struggling member complained: "I can never concentrate on what I'm doing. I cut out dresses, send for writing courses, even sign up for real estate school, but I always drop out and go back to eating full-time." When we're obsessed with overeating, it's difficult to concentrate on losing weight or fully experiencing life. *Food is the great distracter.*

Try practicing the art of concentrating on your eating plan just for today. Focus on the positive aspects of the next twenty-four hours. Don't let your mind become preoccupied or diverted.

Do you have one thing you want to fully experience today? Perhaps you have a mountain to climb, a job you've left half done, or some other interest on which you have not been able to focus your full attention. Maybe you just want to concentrate on improving your self-image.

Whatever you choose, try to concentrate on one thing at a time, and finish what you start.

*Persistence—Stick to It*

A woman died not long ago. She was a wife and mother, only forty-six years old. This woman was no celebrity, and yet her death made the network news. Why? Because she weighed 880 pounds at death, which made her the fattest woman in the world. Eleven firemen carried her on a tarp when she was taken to the hospital with kidney failure.

Simultaneously, another woman was being honored by her diet group for losing more than 100 pounds in a year. What is the difference between these two women? What makes one gain so much and one lose so much? One difference is persistence. Nothing else in the world can take its place. Talent, genius, education, wealth—all of these together are not as helpful as persistence and determination.

Doctors who work with overweight people say motivation may ensure that a person will start a diet, but even the strongest motivation won't predict success. What character trait *will* predict success? Persistence.

No one is trying to tell you persistence is a snap. Interrupting a habit always causes distress because you've stopped doing something you've always done. It's during this time of distress, when the going gets tough, that persistence makes all the difference.

How do you build the ability to persist into your life? Learn to endure the momentary discomforts you may feel, instead of reaching for morsels to soothe the pain away. Sometimes, if you have an emotional pain, you may just have to let it hurt. You can handle that.

The first few days of any new eating regimen—even the healthiest—are usually the time when you need to call up all the persistence you can muster. But don't let up as the pounds come off. Sometimes dieters think they are safe because they are nearing their goal weight. This may be the very time they have to push even harder.

People who have been overweight often find they can *never* stop persisting in their new positive way of eating. Keeping the ability to persevere at a high level is their insurance against slipping back into old, destructive eating patterns.

*Consistency—Live It*

As you lose weight, chances are good that you are also achieving personal inner growth. If so, then you have developed that especially mature discipline, consistency. It is the mark of growth, the capstone of thoughtful change.

Don't mistake disciplined consistency with perfectionism. They have nothing to do with each other. Whenever you say, "Nothing I do is ever good enough," then you are talking about perfectionism, not consistency.

The very word *consistency,* when used in a mature sense, means the freedom to make choices and commitments. The really mature person advances in self-growth based on his or her ability to make commitments, accept responsibilities, and act on them.

*The consistent person has a real contentment.* When you are consistent, you can count on yourself to get you where you know you should go. Consistency, where diet is concerned, usually means the ability to advance in small but steady increments. It marches hand in hand with patience and persistence.

*Staying Power*

You don't have to be Albert Einstein to apply the law of inertia to your weight problem. This law states: *A body remains at rest until a force is applied to it.* Inertia is the quality in matter that resists change.

Inertia sometimes grips us and holds us motionless. We become weighed down with the emotions of being fat, until we cannot move. We sigh and tell ourselves, "Well, I guess I'll just have to learn to live with it." Fortunately, inertia doesn't last forever, and soon we are right back in the same old conflict of being fat and not liking it one bit.

Only one force can cause us to begin again to move toward a thinner, healthier way of life—the force of a positive mind. You've learned now that you *can* change thinking and feeling patterns and behavior. Like the physicist's law, change will occur in direct proportion to the amount of force you apply.

And what you cannot imagine changing for a life-time, you can change for one day. If twenty-four hours is too long a period to even think of going without that extra food, try one hour. Then one hour follows another and another, until you have day after day of healthy eating and its inevitable payoff—weight loss and the thin life.

Learn to *postpone* gratifying the urge to overeat. Then learn to give yourself just as much pleasure from not eating as you used to derive from extra food. You'll have success. And success begets even more success.

*The Great Plateau*

Inertia and discouragement are never so great a problem as when you've hit a weight plateau. What do you do when the diet and exercise that have been working so well for you suddenly stop and you plateau? Here are a few suggestions that may help:

1. Carry a picture of yourself taken when you were slim or a picture of the way you think you'll look.

2. Don't weigh yourself every day. Dieters go through periods when they lose weight slowly. You'll eliminate some of the frustration if you stop hopping on the scale.

3. Check your measurements instead of your weight, as was mentioned previously. If you have been keeping a record, you'll find that your body has been busy reshaping itself even though you haven't lost pounds. Sometimes just knowing that change is occurring can help you get over the emotional trauma of a diet plateau.

4. Go to an extra meeting of your diet group or see your doctor. The doctor will check to see if all your working parts are still in order, or if your diet plan needs a minor adjustment.

If these tonics fail to make the doldrums bearable until the scale continues its downward march, here are some suggestions that can help you jump-start weight loss:

1. Sometimes the temporary removal of flour products will do the trick. Processed flour in breads and pastas are more calorie-dense and quickly absorbed.

2. If water retention becomes a problem, *increase* your water intake by 15 to 20 percent. This will cause diuresis and restart the weight-reduction process.

3. Is your plateau a level of weight where you stayed for any length of time "on the way up"? Your body just may be reluctant to leave an old familiar location. Continued dieting and patience will eventually get you off the plateau.

4. Add a second exercise period or split your exercise time into two periods, one in the morning and one in the evening. Exercising right before a meal can also hasten weight loss.

5. When plateaus persist, check with your doctor to see if you are undergoing any blood chemistry or gastrointestinal disturbances.

6. Last and most important, check to see if you have consciously or unconsciously altered your weight-losing eating plan in any way. You may have to return to keeping a food diary to discover the culprit. Whatever is necessary, *do it*.

Take a look at how far you've come, and then take a minute to be proud of yourself. Just as a plateau in life often results in a turning point, so can a plateau lead to further weight reduction. Be prepared for the good to come.

*Don't Sabotage Your Happiness*

So you've been losing weight, reordering your priorities, and, in general, setting your life straight. Marvelous! Enjoy living today and every day, but be alert to negative thinking, which can come creeping back into your mind when you least expect it.

1. *Watch out* when you begin to think that no matter what you eat you'll never be fat again.

2. *Watch out* when complacency lowers your guard and allows old anger and resentment to reappear.

3. *Watch out* when you find yourself being dishonest about your diet with your friends, your doctor, or yourself.

4. *Watch out* when you become cocky about weight loss.

5. *Watch out* when you drop out of your diet group because you don't need help anymore.

6. *Watch out* when you demand ongoing praise for losing weight.

7. *Watch out* when you become bored with your eating plan and decide to spice it up a bit.

8. *Watch out* when you again attempt to solve any problem with a "little something."

If you come upon these danger signs in your path, quickly reactivate your memory. Remember what your life was like before you found a way of eating to live a healthier, thinner way. Remember going from dark day to dark day without hope.

Danger signs are not meant to run you off the road entirely; they're simply to warn you of bumps ahead. You can then make a choice to go around them or to go straight ahead but with caution.

Many of us have found that, in addition to these danger signs, we need to watch for three other extremes:

1. Never get too bored.
2. Never get too tired.
3. Never get too hungry.

Yet each in its own way, faced positively, could *help* you lose weight.

*Bored*—Two psychology researchers tested overweight students while they performed exceedingly boring or very interesting tasks. They discovered that the students ate far less when they were really interested in what they were doing.

You know that you have eaten to escape boredom. Learning to alternate necessary but boring jobs with tasks you find more intriguing could give you the crucial edge in appetite control.

*Tired*—Getting too tired often becomes an excuse to eat whatever is handy, rather than to prepare foods on your healthy eating plan. Excessive fatigue is also a signal for a quick-energy pick-me-up—which to us means extra food.

Try to alternate periods of heavy energy use with forms of relaxation. Put your feet up for a few minutes, loosen your clothing, close your eyes, and breathe deeply. They'll be minutes well spent. Don't try to fool yourself that you don't have the time. It will take a lot longer to quit work for a bout of overeating just because you got too tired.

*Hungry*—If you allow yourself to get so busy that you delay your regular mealtime, you can get so hungry that the meal you have won't fill you up and you could reach for extra calories.

## Take Charge of Cravings

Is there one certain food over which you seem to have no control? Over the years, diet-club members have reported that specific foods (mostly of the sweet and high-fat variety) were beyond their ability to handle. These foods, called "binge foods," were ones in which one bite was too much and the whole package not nearly enough.

"I can't have anything chocolate in the house," said one self-styled chocoholic. "Even if I have it locked in a kitchen cupboard out of sight, it sings to me until I answer."

If you have a binge food that powerful, whatever it is, simply don't keep it around. That doesn't mean you can never again have a bite of this food. It does mean you'll have to wait until more positive things have become sweeter to you than any chocolate drop.

It is a paradox that we overeaters fall in love with certain foods. Most of us have tales of sick bodies and unhappy lives brought about, in part, because of our dependence on these binge foods. And yet, year after year we have surrounded our favorite foods with a mystique which gives them magical and even curative powers.

*The only thing we get from binge food is fat.*

Learn to recognize the storm warnings your body sends to your mind, warnings that have, in the past, sent you straight to your binge foods. You can control your physical cravings by not taking that first bite.

Certain foods can be triggers to overeat, but certain times and circumstances can be as well. For example, you may be a night eater. Many overweight people consume the bulk of their calories after six o'clock in the evening, almost guaranteeing the calories will go straight to their fat cells. Some are unable to sleep without a full stomach, and still others awaken in the night and remain insomniac until they have satisfied their night craving.

If you have this problem (or if you have periodic cravings of any kind), you can try some of these strategies:

1. Keep a bottle of water at your bedside.

2. Ask your physician to check you for low blood sugar levels—hypoglycemia—which may be keeping you awake and hungry.

3. Save a piece of fruit from your eating plan and eat it before going to bed. Fruit contains fructose and insulin isn't necessary in its metabolism, so a hypoglycemic reaction is less likely.

4. Ask yourself if night eating compensates for a lack of sexual activity or a nagging task left undone.

5. Discuss the use of a temporary sedative with your doctor.

6. Take a hot shower before going to bed.

Deep-seated habits require you to be ingenious, so try anything that sounds reasonable to change your time-related eating behavior. You can do it, if you believe you can.

Other time-related factors, often brought about by natural changes in your body's chemistry, can make craving food a problem. During the premenstrual period, many women crave sweets. This craving doesn't last long—usually one day—but it can play havoc with your eating plan.

If you have PMS, you'll want to satisfy this craving without consuming too many empty sugar calories.

Practice relaxation techniques, says Dr. Carl L. Ebnother, who equates sweet craving with premenstrual tension. Self-hypnosis, meditation, or exercise can relieve the tension and along with it, the craving.

If you have a premenstrual craving for sweets or an abnormal craving at any other time, talk to your doctor, especially if you discover you can't handle it by yourself. Don't ignore the problem. It can set you up for unnecessary weight gain and reinforce old eating habits. That's how we gained excess weight in the first place.

*Wrong Time, Wrong Place*

Other times and places often challenge our new healthy eating plans. Holidays and vacations are the worst. We tend to define *vacation* as a time to take a break from everything. What we often forget is that, no matter how far away we go, we can't leave behind our firm commitment to a healthy lifestyle. "I decided to forget about my diet during my vacation," said a dieter, retelling a too-familiar story. "I ate my way clear across the country and had to buy a new dress, in a bigger size, to wear home."

You can't take a vacation from a healthful way of eating, because your craving for excess food never goes on vacation. Your vacation isn't a two-week binge. It's a time to get away from your surroundings, your job, or school. It's a time to relax and recharge your coping batteries.

Let go of the idea that the only fun in living comes from eating. You can have more real fun sticking to your good-living diet than by eating any amount of rich, high-calorie treats. "Having to buy new clothes just so I could get home ruined my vacation," remembers the woman who ate her way across the country. "When I think about it, I only remember how angry I was with myself."

The great and wonderful things you desire will not come easy. When you are on vacation, you may be tempted to return to your old destructive ways. Don't do it, or you will have a vacation to remember, all right. It just won't be a very happy memory.

The same is true of many holidays we celebrate. Often, our celebrations revolve around feasts. And during holidays, overeating is sanctioned by everyone. We're told every year, "Oh, you can't diet on Thanksgiving." In the past, we happily agreed. But now, we know what we really want.

This Thanksgiving, give thanks for the food you *don't* eat. That's the only way an overeater can truly celebrate. "I can't take a holiday from my compulsion to overeat," says one dieter. "One Christmas, I casually decided I could handle some sweet desserts I hadn't eaten for over a year. It was five months and forty-two pounds later before I came off that binge."

Just because you've decided that healthy eating is the way you are going to live your life, don't think parties, holidays, or family gatherings won't be any fun. Here's the real fun of holidays: getting on the scales the next day and seeing that you've held your weight; feeling no overeating guilt; keeping your hard-won self-esteem; knowing at last what really makes you happy. "The year I followed my eating plan despite the holiday atmosphere," says the woman who once gained forty-two pounds, "was the first year I truly enjoyed and concentrated on Christmas."

*Don't Fool Yourself*

In addition to all the diet challenges found on our calendar, there are times in every dieter's day when five little words can spell disaster. Ever catch yourself in one of these rationalizations?

*One little bite won't hurt.* It's the most common and deadly dieter's excuse of all, because it sounds so true. What harm could one little bite possibly do? The answer is, a lot. One bite doesn't add a lot of calories, but it does break down your ability to control the next bite and the next. "I never meant to eat the whole cake," said one diet club member. "I just slivered it to death."

Psychologists who specialize in modifying eating behavior know that each time you take a bite, you weaken yourself for the next time. But behavior cuts both ways. Each time you don't eat when you want to, you're stronger the next time.

*I'll make it up tomorrow.* The food you overeat today is not magically canceled out by what you don't eat tomorrow. It is impossible to predict twenty-four hours in advance what your mood will be and whether, by some superhuman effort, you'll be able to eat even less than your diet plan calls for.

*To hell with diets anyway.* Most overeaters use this defiant excuse after they've already taken that first bite. They rationalize: "I've blown it, so I might as well go all the way."

But think a minute. There's a great deal of difference between a 50-calorie bite and a 500-calorie helping. And don't kid yourself that you don't care. Later, you'll care very much. Then your guilt could drive you back to the refrigerator for a real binge!

Those "five little words" are hidden deceivers. They tell us what we may want to hear for the moment—not the facts. But we can get rid of false rationalizations by recognizing them for what they are.

Remember, after you get rid of "one little bite won't hurt," "I'll make it up tomorrow," and "to hell with diets anyway," there *are* five little words you can live by. They're what this book is all about—*one day at a time*—the way you truly want to live.

Winning the weight game requires that we control our cravings each day, all day. One dieter reported to her group: "When I found my hand reaching for an unneeded dessert, I talked to myself out loud. 'You don't want that! You really want something better for your body.'" Instead of giving in, time after time, day after day, learn to be firm in your refusal. You know how to do this.

The philosopher John Stuart Mill said that we should "learn to seek our happiness by limiting our desires, rather than attempting to satisfy them." He could have been speaking directly to those of us who try to satisfy every desire with food. How many times have you overeaten because you were disappointed, or didn't attract the right person, or didn't get the job, or didn't get the recognition you deserved? But that was before you found your way back to health.

We overeaters often act impulsively on passion rather than on a well-thought-out action plan. We *are* passionate people. We have strong drives, diverse appetites, and deep feelings. But the planned-action side of our nature is often not fully developed.

Develop your ability to plan and then to act responsibly on that plan. Practice saying no to your desire for excess food and yes to your desire for a healthy, slender body. The more you practice, the easier it will be.

Not giving in to desires has become as much of a habit as satisfying them used to be. Saying no has weakened your desire to eat and strengthened your new desire to live without excess food. You're finding it's not as hard to say no to extra food as it once was.

*Learn to Forgive Yourself*

"You won't believe this," said the tearful newcomer to the diet group, "but I gained four pounds today. During the last year I've gained thirty-six and I dieted most of the year! I can't imagine what I would weigh if I hadn't.

"It seems food is the only source of enjoyment I have. But every day, with every pound gained, I'm more unhappy. And I'm scared, too. Where will it end? I consumed 20,000 calories one day—I counted them—and I still didn't quit. I just kept stuffing."

The members of this young woman's diet group not only believed her story, but they, each in turn, got up and told similar ones. "I thought I was the only one who did such crazy things with food," the newcomer said after the meeting. "I see I'm not alone, and I believe if you can do it, so can I."

If you are an on-again, off-again dieter, the fear of failure can prevent you from giving yourself another chance to succeed. Some people have resorted to desperate acts to ensure success—from having their jaws wired together to going on Gandhi-like fasts. Why? Because they desperately fear failure if left on their own.

If you're slimming down a day at a time and never take a wayward bite, that's fabulous. But if you do err, know that each day is a new chance you can give yourself. It doesn't matter what you ate yesterday. Today you are committing yourself anew to following your healthful eating plan.

Making this commitment each morning will free you from the fear of failure and allow you to concentrate on the positive things in your day—the composure that comes when you're working for the image you've always wanted, the confusion that leaves your daily life when you follow a disciplined way of eating. Your mind will not be clouded by the effects of too much high-calorie food. You will see self-confidence replace fear. One by one your problems will become manageable. You will not be depressed about your weight because you can honestly say, *"I'm doing something about it."*

As you progress on your new eating plan, know that you may always have some limitations. If you want to avoid a slip, stay out of slippery places. The payoff for such caution is obvious. You will be far less likely to stray from the plan of eating you've chosen to mold your new body.

But what if you do slip off your plan, despite your best intentions? The most important thing for you to remember is not to punish yourself for a slip by more overeating. Be thankful that you have heard the warning bell, that at last you have an overpowering urge to move toward wholeness and health. Try to see the thin person who you really are. Set your sights on becoming that person on the outside as well as on the inside.

If you slip, forgive yourself immediately. Set yourself free from any need for further self-punishment. In that way you can start again with a clean slate, without any hold-over guilt. Sure you'll have problems—that's part of being a sensitive human being in a complex world. But no known illness, economic disaster, or personal trouble has yet been cured by massive doses of chocolate. Setting simple goals and backing them up with careful contingency planning is a good way for you to face the challenges of living day by day.

## Emotions

When we look in the mirror and see the extra pounds on our bodies, it doesn't occur to us that some of those pounds have names like *envy, disappointment, jealousy,* and *hatred.*

Did you once overeat because someone had a bigger house, received your coveted promotion, married your girl- or boyfriend? Of course you did. The big troubles, the bitter disappointments, the deep wrongs—all the tragedies of our lives hang on our bodies. If you are ever to lose weight and keep it off, you need to let go of even the most heartbreaking sorrow, even the greatest wrong. If you keep them in your heart and mind, you risk keeping the pounds that go with them.

The most common emotions that affect overeaters are anger, loneliness, guilt, fear, anxiety, and depression. While dealing with these emotions, we frequently have trouble controlling food quantity and nibble all day on unhealthy foods we associate with comfort.

How can you deal with the temptation to overeat when difficult emotions arise?

1. Identify what's behind your emotion and then accept and experience the emotion as a natural reaction rather than trying to dull it with food.

2. Minimize the opportunities you have to eat impulsively by keeping busy in some challenging activity. In other words, don't brood; get busy.

3. Watch the amounts and kinds of food you eat, changing from processed snack foods to fresh vegetables and fruits.

Now let's take some specific emotions, see how they affect your eating plan, and identify what you can do to stay on the right path.

*Anger*

Anger is an extremely destructive emotion. Because overweight people are often stereotyped as "jolly," it may surprise some to know that psychologists consider anger to be one of our outstanding character traits. But we experience anger differently: Our anger isn't acted out against others, it's acted out against ourselves.

Have you ever been so angry at someone you binged just to "show" them? Have you ever gotten so angry about something that you overate out of spite? Of course you have. But worse yet, you have angrily overeaten without even knowing it. If anger is passive and remains unexpressed, it soaks up vital energy and eventually causes depression and added pounds.

Most of us don't want to show anger, so we bottle it up inside. We try to put on such a good face for the world. We hold our legitimate anger inside until it explodes in one big angry eating binge. The trouble with taking out anger on our bodies is that we don't solve our problems, and we create new and probably worse problems.

To grow on an emotional level, we need to learn to use anger in a creative way. Anger is really just undirected energy. If you direct it outward at your problem (instead of internalizing it), you can use this energy to find solutions.

If you're angry with specific people, try this: Write the names of the people you're angry with on a "grudge list," then decide why you hold them within this circle of resentment. Ask yourself: Has my life been made better for this anger? The point is that holding on to anger stops us from growing. And it doesn't seem to matter if your anger is righteous. It's best to let go of all anger as quickly as possible.

Take a good look at the "grudge list" you've just written. Is there anyone or anything on it worth gaining weight over? Is there anyone on your list who would change for the better if you gained more weight? Of course not.

Anger has another solution. Try writing your frustration away. If someone has angered you until you are unhappy (and hungry), sit down and write a letter to that person. Explain exactly what you think about his or her behavior. Really lay it on. Now, put the letter away for twenty-four hours.

The next day, retrieve your letter and read it again with renewed satisfaction. Now, sit down and write yourself a letter *from the other person.* While wearing the other person's shoes, write out the problems that have him or her baffled and furious.

Read both letters again. You don't have as much satisfaction in your first one, do you? Finally, tear them both up and throw them away. Nobody's hurt, your frustration's gone, and you probably have a deeper insight into your own and the other person's feelings than you had before.

It is plain that a life spent holding deep anger or even several petty resentments is an unhappy, futile life. And if you happen to be an overeater, it means that feeding this negative emotion will make you fatter and angrier. Remember each day that anger is the most destructive thing you can do to yourself. You're much too busy for anger. You've got a beautiful life to live and work to do.

*Loneliness*

For some, overeating is a search for the end of loneliness. And it's true that for a moment overeating can block out your aloneness. But the feeling returns when the eating binge ends.

Almost daily, we experience losses that leave us feeling lonely and rejected. We lose a job, move from one home to another, get a divorce, or simply misplace our billfold. We aren't invited to a social event, a friend is unavailable, a lover fails to call. For overeaters, each loss, small or large, can throw us into an overeating binge in an effort to cope with the loneliness and rejection we feel.

What is the antidote? Love yourself more. When you love yourself, you'll have no need to fill your empty spaces with extra fat and sugar.

Perhaps your fear of rejection has caused you to unconsciously adopt behavior and attitudes that actually bring about rejection. To cover up your fear, you may display an attitude of aloofness toward people. They, in turn, think you're a snob.

How can you get over your fear of rejection? Start by recognizing attitudes you have that invite rejection. Think before you speak, because old habits of responding are hard to break. Finally, recognize that you are not alone in your problem. Nearly everyone feels rejection at times, even people whose bodies are thin.

You used to depend on overeating for relief from rejection and loneliness. Food picked you up when you were down. It made you feel less lonely and unloved for a brief moment, but then it dropped you very low.

Now you're finished with a false dependence on food. You've begun to develop abilities that can safely bring you through any problem.

*Guilt*

We overeaters, with few exceptions, have become the rocket scientists of guilt: guilt because of the times we promised others we'd lose weight and didn't, guilt for all the times we promised ourselves we were going to stop overeating and didn't. Sometimes we feel guilty for just being alive and less than perfect. For us, guilt is the mother of all negative emotions.

Guilt is often the subject of support groups that deal with the feelings lying behind overeating. "We are people who can't let go of guilt over the least thing," explains one member, "without first punishing ourselves for the transgression. Our punishment finds its expression in overeating."

Many of us overweight people carry a load of unnecessary guilt around with us. But we learn to travel lighter as we thin down because we lose the need to punish ourselves for being fat.

When you become conscious that your guilty feelings have no basis in reality, try to remember that excess guilt is often the product of a highly sensitive nature. You can turn the ability to feel deeply into an asset. Truly sensitive people, when they rid themselves of guilt, become the kind of people others seek out for advice.

Here are some other suggestions to help you overcome paralyzing guilt:

1. Analyze your reasons for feeling guilty. Then forgive yourself for past wrongs and move on.

2. Don't brood over failures or assume an excessive burden of guilt for them. See where mistakes were made, resolve them, avoid repeating them, and then forget them.

3. Look at your guilt for what it is—an act of self-indulgence. *Are you using guilt as an excuse for standing still in your life?*

4. Ask yourself if you enjoy guilt. Does guilt make you feel more important?

Successful adults with positive emotional attitudes

recognize guilt and get rid of it. Write about your guilt on a piece of paper. Then tear it up in little pieces or burn it. This helps to dramatize the idea of ridding yourself of guilty feelings, real or imagined. Now, you're done with it for good.

Of course, one of the best ways to be guilt-free is to prevent guilt in the first place. When you have done or said something that bothers your conscience, admit it to yourself and to the other person involved, and then *make it right*. You will feel better instantly and this action will squash guilt before it starts.

## Fear

Sometimes we overeaters are fearful, and that makes us great worriers. Deep inside we carry little seeds of self-doubt from which all worry sprouts. This sense of insecurity creates emotional tensions so that worry can actually become a safety valve.

Franklin D. Roosevelt consoled the nation in the 1930s economic depression by saying, "The only thing we have to fear is fear itself." Overweight people, who are sometimes in a different kind of depression, could say the same about worry: *The only thing we have to worry about is worry itself.*

Worry—about the future, about failure, about a thousand imaginary or actual problems—is one of the greatest obstacles to creating and maintaining your thin, healthy life. And it certainly doesn't do much for your peace of mind, either.

Worry and fear go hand in hand. Neither solves a problem, but they do work to break you down both physically and emotionally, making anything you attempt more difficult.

For some, worry becomes such a way of life, they block their own progress. They paralyze themselves by obsessing on the question, "Will I measure up?" For worrying, fearful people, the most ready answer is, "I'll protect myself and not even try."

You can rid yourself of unreasonable worry by understanding fully that you alone determine your future. Other people cannot control you unless you allow them to. The next twenty-four hours are in your hands to do with as you will. You can build the positive power to eliminate worry and build optimism.

Admit to yourself that you worry because, deep inside, you feel lost. Insecurity often results from thinking too much without *putting thoughts into action.* When you procrastinate, you live in a state of perpetual frustration. You come to doubt your goals and lose confidence in your own abilities.

The way out of this trap is to form an adequate sense of inner security. Have faith in yourself. Then swing into action.

And don't be overconcerned. This can intensify fear. Remember, reasonable fears are a natural and normal response to living. Many of us fear the unknown future, but most of those fears never materialize.

Try to put fear in perspective. Sometimes we dramatize our lives: everything becomes a catastrophic tragedy, when in reality most ordinary fears are merely inconveniences. Perhaps you are trying to be perfect. You can work yourself into an absolute frenzy when you place this burden on yourself. Learn to relax and lower your perfectionistic expectations, and fear will be greatly reduced.

Yet, at times real anxiety overtakes us. Our lives seem to be floating on a sea of meaninglessness. Sometimes our response to this depressive feeling is frantic activity; at other times, withdrawal. We are particularly good at withdrawing, because we never withdraw alone. Food goes with us.

When anxiety drags you down and you feel a depressive sense of detachment from the world, the best medicine is to seek out support from others. Call up a dear friend, doctor, or clergy, and try to talk your fears out before you act on them. Try to share experiences. Feelings of fellowship will grow out of honest sharing. And remember to return what is given to you. If someone shows you warmth, acknowledge it and respond to it in kind. Be sensitive to the overtures of others and they, in turn, will be sensitive to yours. Anxiety breeds on supposed rejection, when it could be only a lack of appreciation.

One of the biggest anxieties we struggle with, and one of the most common reasons for diet failure, is a simple fear of hunger. Because most of us have eaten whenever we felt real or imagined hunger, we fear that not feeding the sensation of hunger is impossible. Whenever we tried in the past to control eating bouts between meals, the fear of hunger has gripped us until we were compelled to eat again.

These anxiety attacks are real, but they can be stopped. Try arresting your anxiety by scolding it: "Stop that this minute!" or "Start behaving yourself!"

Many people find that this causes the anxiety to weaken or disappear. Although this sounds like a very simple-minded technique, telling your unreasonable anxiety to "Stop that!" is worth a try, and it may be all that's necessary.

After all, if you have eaten a full meal only to find yourself, after an hour, driven to eat by the fear of hunger, it is safe to assume that you are not on the verge of starvation.

How do such anxieties start? Parents, teachers, peers, television advertisements, and society in general are all makers of hunger myths. The most important thing for us is to know how to confront these hunger fears.

*Depression*

Overweight people can become very depressed. We feel "down" or "blue" or "in the dumps" when we are having problems following our eating plan.

There are no magic cures for the diet blues, but there are some practical ideas for overcoming mild depression so that you don't abandon yourself and can quickly get back to the fun of living.

Mild diet depression is simply the conviction of one's own helplessness. Once you begin to think of yourself as an effective, in-charge human being, you cease being depressed.

In cases like this, the mood of depression is not too intense and does not require professional help. Self-help can often work. Here are some blues-busters:

*Get moving.* Depressed people have a tendency to wallow in their negativity and become lethargic. Try not to color everything black; remember the things that give you joy and get up and do something. Depression may melt away when your mind and body become active.

*Fight against helplessness.* Achieve something. Do something you know you're good at. As you achieve some satisfaction, you will naturally exert more control over your life. It's just like learning to walk. After the first few timid steps, you're off and running.

*Talk it out.* Find a friend with a patient, supportive ear—maybe someone in your diet support group—and simply talk it out. Sharing feelings can work wonders. When you're through, you feel as though a weight is lifted and you feel less alone. Be careful, however, to avoid dwelling on your depression story. Endlessly repeating your problems can alienate friends and increase your focus on your depression, making you feel worse. Once you've aired your feelings, let them go.

In some cases, you may find yourself battling depression that goes beyond the "diet blues." If the above suggestions don't seem to help, if you just can't pull yourself out of "the black hole," consider seeking professional help. A good therapist can gently help you find the sources of and solutions to some of your most difficult struggles.

You may also want to reread this section on depression from time to time. It's important for you to arm yourself with some action steps against the times when you are "down in the dumps." What you are doing—building a life that is healthier, happier, and thinner—is much too important to be left to chance. It's more than a hobby; it's the key to peace and well-being. It's survival.

*Stress*

Stress is a condition influenced chiefly by outside forces in combination with inside emotions. Though not an emotion itself, stress is a dangerous threat to achieving and maintaining weight loss and health. It can be a tension- and anxiety-producing force that pushes us to overeat.

We all undergo stress in our everyday lives. A certain amount of it keeps us moving. Stress, in a constructive sense, can even provide challenges for us. But too much stress and pressure is likely to cause us real suffering. Though we may seem peaceful on the surface, inside we can be churning with conflict.

Stress is the enemy of everyone trying to control food

intake and build a more healthful life. Too much stress can manifest itself in nervousness, sleeplessness, irritability, inability to concentrate, and even loss of muscle coordination.

Since food is a means of relieving tension for many overweight people, it's going to be harder to diet during stress periods such as the following:

1. After the death or serious illness of a family member.

2. When looking for or starting a new job.

3. During marital problems.

4. Just before or after moving.

5. While in financial difficulty.

There are times when pressure builds. Pressure, like a spring, is just wound-up energy. If you don't jump off at the right time, you can hit the ceiling.

The good news is that there are many ways to deal with these feelings of pressure. Most of us used to overeat, but that is no longer the way we want to handle stress. We have to find an escape valve less destructive than food.

You can always read a book, lose yourself in a movie, or work on your hobby. There's nothing high-calorie about those simple tension relievers. But sometimes we need more. If we find ourselves reaching a boiling point, then we'd better take action.

Don't bottle stressful feelings up. Try talking them out. Many times others can help with a problem that has you climbing the walls.

Try getting out of yourself, devoting energy instead to a purpose or cause. This takes your mind away from yourself.

Don't sulk at home with old hurts. Get out, relax, and have fun. Relaxation absorbs pressure like a sponge.

It might even be a good idea to hang this sign some-where in your mind: *Having fun is essential to my emotional health.*

Here are other tension-relieving techniques that help you cope with everyday pressure:

1. *Take a short nap.* Children take naps to restore energy, why not you? Even ten minutes will help.

2. *Keep telling yourself you are relaxed.* If you tell yourself often enough, you eventually will be.

3. *Learn to forgive.* Hatred and resentment cause more tension than any other emotions.

4. *Pretend you are happy.* Act as if you are happy and you will grow into the role.

5. *Learn to laugh more.* Pressure subsides when you stop taking yourself so seriously.

6. *Keep in contact with things that inspire you.* If this means carrying poetry in your wallet or pinning weight-losing slogans to your refrigerator, so be it. Refuse to be grim.

The most important thing for your health and life, without exception, is learning to live—and live well—without excess food.

### Dealing with Emotions

Too many times we reached for extra calories because we needed something to quiet anxieties or banish stress. Somehow we thought food was the only cure for the lump in our throats. It wasn't.

In our old life, stress created tension, and prolonged tension made it impossible to follow a disciplined way of eating. We can't live that way and achieve our desires.

### Learn to Relax

A very simple way to relax, reduce stress, and elimi-nate anxiety is just a breath away. Experts recommend a simple yet powerful relaxation technique: deep breathing. Breathing is one of the easiest things in life to control—you can slow or speed it up at will. Try deep-breathing slowly from your diaphragm, right now; pause for a moment after inhaling, and then exhale completely. While you're breathing, consciously allow your shoulder muscles to relax. Do this exercise again and again each day. To remind yourself, associate deep breathing with some common activity such as checking the time. Each time you look at the clock, inhale deeply, then continue with what you need to do, a little more relaxed.

If you have a tape recorder, get a blank tape and record the following statements in a soothing voice. If you don't have a recorder, write them on a sheet of paper. Play back or read aloud these suggestions when you feel yourself becoming tense:

1. You are a calm person.
2. You avoid worry about things you can't change.
3. You have control over negative feelings.
4. You avoid stressful situations.
5. You avoid tension-producing people.
6. You are breathing deeply and regularly.
7. You are seeing yourself as thin, fit, and healthy.
8. You think of yourself as a person with self-control.
9. You are able to relax completely.
10. You trust yourself.

After you have listened to your own voice outlining these positive ideas, you are ready to try some mental imagery. Imagine yourself in an unavoidable situation or argument that produces a lot of tension for you. But this time, instead of reacting stressfully, watch yourself playing the part of a poised, calm, and relaxed person. Practice this exercise whenever you feel tension that might cause you to reach for a food pacifier. In a short time, you'll be more relaxed, and eventually you'll weigh less.

Exercise is also a great stress reducer. If you're jumpy about anything at all, walk around the block. And while you're at it, use your positive power to imagine new friends, fabulous parties, a wonderful job, looking thin and healthy, and a closet full of new clothes in a smaller size. According to Dr. Richard Driscoll, a psychologist at Eastern State Psychiatric Hospital in Tennessee, the combination of exercise and pleasant thoughts helps banish anxiety.

*Release Your Emotions*

Unpleasant emotions are accompanied by tightness in the skeletal muscles and the muscles of the internal organs. Keep up this muscle-tensing long enough and you begin to hurt.

The stomach is one of the primary organs afflicted by negative emotions. When the stomach muscles tighten because of emotional upheaval, the feeling is that of a lump in the upper abdomen; some people describe it as a "stone." When the stomach muscles squeeze down really hard, a pain is produced, sometimes a very severe one, which can feel a lot like ulcer pain. How is this pain translated by overeaters? "I'm hungry," they think. "I'd better eat a little something."

It's obvious you've been looking for peace of mind— that quest is universal. But you have been looking for it in all the wrong places—the refrigerator, the fast food restaurant, and the candy machine. Remember, it's not what *happens* to you that creates problems, but how you *react* to your life situation—are you victim or master?

One of the best ways to train yourself to react with positive power is to communicate with yourself. You've seen that it pays to talk to others about your feelings; now, talk to yourself.

When you are exasperated, worried, or depressed over any emergency—big or small—say to yourself:

> *I am not responsible for all that happens to me, but I am responsible for how I react emotionally. I will not become disturbed and blow this problem out of proportion. Excessive concern only causes me to be tired and tense.*
>
> *I must remember that I feel better physically and mentally when I choose to be cheerful and self-encouraging. I have perfect control over my thoughts and emotions. I can make them as positive and helpful as I want.*
>
> *No one else can upset me or tie me up in emotional knots if I refuse to allow it.*

Adapt this script to specific situations. For example, if your spouse, boss, neighbor, or friend makes you angry, mention this person by name in your self-communication. It will allow you to focus your positive thought and block negative emotional activity.

### Harness Positive Emotions

If we're not careful, our emotions can rule us. That is why it's necessary to find a way to use them constructively instead of destructively.

Every day of your new life, you are harnessing your emotional energy for positive ends. Instead of allowing your negative emotions to enervate you, use your positive emotional energy. Love is human energy in its most positive form. Love life enough to give it to yourself, now and in the future.

Let your emotions show in creative ways. Your feelings play an important role in your creative life. Don't hesitate to express them. Say "thank you" for the smallest gift. Share the tears of someone with a disappointment. Don't keep your praise to yourself.

With such positive energy forces, you will make good decisions about how to proceed in all your life. The disastrous forces of hate, criticism, resentment, jealousy, and self-pity will wither from disuse. You will empty yourself of everything you don't need.

You are the only person who can activate this positive energy force. No one, no matter how much they may want to, can do this for you. But once you have decided to use love and other positive emotions in your life, you will discover you have made a space in your heart for everything you need. It's important for your mind, body, and spirit. An old Yiddish story has God asking you only one question: "Why didn't you become you?"

## Up Against the Wall

Always remember what it's like to be fat. First there are the constant fears: of ridicule, social disapproval, being lectured, and not getting the job, friend, or relationship we want. Is it any wonder if we grow "thin-skinned" under our burden of flesh?

Then there is the loneliness of being different from others, and even worse, of being different from the person we want to be.

There is misery, discrimination, recrimination—and we end by rejecting ourselves.

We've learned the lessons of being fat all too well. When it comes time to learn to be thin, to live in a healthy new, creative way, the experience is alien to us.

### What Is It Like to Be Thin?

You will touch the earth lightly; nothing will rattle or shake as you pass by. You will be able to pay attention to the world outside your body; every mirror will stop reflecting defeat. You will not have to hold your opinions or talent back, trading opportunity for acceptance.

Alone will not be as lonely, because you will be with an inner friend who is helpful. You will be in balance with life. Food will have a place, but not every place.

You will wake and find your dream of losing weight is real. You will believe that it is for good this time. You will feel quiet inside, a kind of rich silence too many calories stifled.

We overeaters have lived in a fat world separated from the world we longed for by one act, one moment of decision. Our world was often filled with unloving, hostile people, a world devoid of empathy and compassion, a world of suffering and despair. Escape didn't seem possible. When we struggled against our place in that world, we were laughed at or scorned.

We walked down streets avoiding the eyes of oncoming people, because sometimes we could see disgust mirrored there—their own and ours. On occasion, because of a pressing inner need, we would reach out our hand, only to draw it back, empty.

*Then we made a decision.* We would take charge of our lives—controlling our eating and not being controlled by it—from this day forward. We would grow mentally and emotionally and take our rightful place with mature people.

By this act of decision, a new world was created. Where before we saw and felt only pain, we now saw the world as our opportunity. Where before we saw disgust, now we saw admiration. Where before we saw only eating as a solution, now we saw limitless options. Where before we came away empty-handed, now we had another hand in ours.

Had the world really changed that much or had we changed?

*If you want to change your world, first change yourself.*

### The Point of No Return

Hope for the point of no return. Hope that today will be the day you become unalterably committed to a life without excess food, to a body unburdened with extra calories to burn, to a mind and heart free to explore the new.

This is your life. You're unwilling to spend one more day of it in turmoil. Go beyond the point of no return and become unwilling to turn back. The old way of using food to fuel emotional hunger cannot offer you peace or joy. The new life you seek can offer you all this and more.

Hope for the point of no return. Beyond that point, it will be easier for you to go ahead than it will be to turn back. Take some time now to question your life and correct anything that could block your physical and emotional plans to change your life. Ask yourself these questions:

1. Have I chosen to eat for maximum health with such conviction that there is no going back?

2. Have I changed from negative to positive thinking, forever finished with self-hate?

3. Have I grown in self-esteem so that I can walk proudly and look anyone in the eye?

4. Am I confidently living one day at a time, searching for serenity and peace of mind?

5. Am I reaching out for added strength to other overeaters who are winning over their problem?

6. Do I have firm hope that a better life lies ahead of me?

7. Am I controlling my emotions without letting them control me?

8. Have I fully accepted that I have a lifetime eating problem, which can be overcome with a lifetime positive living program?

9. Am I searching for serenity and peace of mind?

10. Do I accept that inner growth must keep pace with weight loss?

11. Am I honest with myself in all things?

By self-questioning and deeply probing our minds, we keep ourselves headed in the right direction and remind ourselves where we came from. Deep down in your heart, you find the answer: control over food.

To maintain the weight you've worked so hard to achieve, you need real growth from the inside out and a balance in all things. You need to use some of your tremendous fighting energy to continue becoming who you want to be. You are no longer battling *against*, but fighting *for*. This is your positive goal.

Formerly, all the food you could eat left you hungry. When you have the slender, healthy body you want and are in charge of your eating, you will truly know fulfillment.

# Introduction to Book II

*I*n the first half of *The Thin Books*, you quit playing the waiting game and carefully crafted a personal program to attain the weight and body shape that is natural for you. You formed a healthy eating, exercise, and positive attitude program to last a lifetime. You learned successful strategies and skills that will help you create a life with style.

Yet, life is lived one day at a time, and every overweight person starts the day with one question: How can I get going and keep going?

Action is key. It helps you see each day as a challenge and puts you in charge of your day, 365 days a year. It keeps you on track, and it keeps your goal in sight.

The second half of this book consists of easy-to-use daily meditations designed to combat negative "failure talk" and keep you on the expressway to success. In these meditations, you will use twelve principles of action to help you energize every day. The principles are intended to overlap each other, so that when you focus on one, you automatically improve in all the others. Write them on a piece of paper and post them where you will see them often. Then assimilate them through the meditations; they will change your life forever.

## The Twelve Principles of Personal Action
1. Develop a solid understanding of your unique worth.
2. Practice confidence every day.

3. Radiate warmth.
4. Learn what your fears are.
5. Acknowledge a burning desire to be thin and healthy.
6. Make your own sunlight.
7. Take charge of your life.
8. Do whatever needs to be done *now.*
9. Take weight loss in steps.
10. Reject rejection firmly and totally.
11. Don't fight inevitable change.
12. Play life to win.

You'll find that these principles don't wear out with constant use; in fact, the harder you use them, the more relevant they become. These twelve principles empower you to do what you want to do most. Can you imagine what they will do for your self-esteem?

As we have learned, it's not enough to think positive thoughts. Positive thoughts need action to transform them into accomplishments. In the following pages, you'll find a course of daily action to lead you to your desired weight and, ultimately, to your life goals.

No one limits your success but you. If you want to be more and learn more today, then *do* more today. By adding an action meditation to your daily routine, you will be taking the specific steps that lead you straight to the winner's circle.

## January 1           The Shape of Things to Come

*Enough, if something from our hands have power*
*To live, and act, and serve the future hour.*
                    *—William Wordsworth*

A new year stretches ahead, and you have the power in your hands to make a fresh beginning today. This is the day you're going to begin looking and feeling like the person you want to be, the day you're going to make the word *action* the most important word in your vocabulary. Why? Because you have made a positive decision about yourself, for today and all your future days.

But don't stop at decision making. Decision without action is like living in a house with no windows. Open your house to the light by putting your decision into action. Decide on an eating and exercise plan that will help you lose weight healthfully. Then reread the principles of the action plan in the introduction. Today, just become familiar with them. Try them on. If they fit, make them your own.

Today, start the process of making action a part of your daily life.

*Today's Action Plan: Right where I am, from whatever weight or point of despair, I will make a positive start on my future.*

*Repeat—iterate, reiterate, reproduce, echo, re-echo, drum, hammer, redouble, begin again, resume, return to.*

—Roget's Thesaurus

Repetition is the mother's milk of fat-free living. Repeating an action makes it part of you, whether it's habitually choosing a healthful meal or reinforcing a life-changing decision day after day.

But you must use *effective* repetition, not distracted, mindless singsong. That means you must read it, write it, speak it, listen to it, and then take action and *do* it. You must repeat a positive action until it dances in your head.

Repetition is a major ingredient of success. If you're not taking positive action right now, today, you won't be able to reinforce that act later on. The entire reason for repeating an action in the first place is to insert it into your new positive lifestyle.

Today, practice repetition. Reinforcing a good habit puts you in training to become a winner!

*Today's Action Plan: With every breath I take, I will repeat the idea that the healthful life is worth reinforcing.*

*When the fight begins within himself, a man's worth something.*

—*Robert Browning*

The first principle in your action plan says, "Develop a solid understanding of your unique worth." What does that mean? You can answer that question for yourself.

Some people project an unmistakable stamp of self-worth. Their presence is a powerful force. They reflect a sense of unique individuality that is beyond physical beauty or even good grooming. "What have they got that I haven't?" you ask. They have self-pride, the honest pride that comes from capitalizing on one's own potential.

You're cheating yourself if you don't believe in your unique worth. You're living life at a lower level than you deserve. Convince yourself that you're worth your greatest effort and you won't have to try to convince other people. They'll know it.

Today, accept the worthiness of yourself. You have a right to a thinner, healthier body.

*Today's Action Plan: When I walk through a door, I will radiate the unmistakable look of my unique worth. I will be a presence.*

## January 4 — The Ingredients of Friendship

*A friend is one to whom you may pour out all the contents of your heart, chaff and grain together, knowing that the gentlest of hands will take and sift it, keep what is worth keeping, and with a breath of kindness, blow the rest away.*

*—Arabian proverb*

We expect six qualities from our friends. We want them to *keep our confidences* and *share their loyalty, warmth, affection, supportiveness,* and *sense of humor.* Is this what you bring to your best friend—yourself? Do you stand up for yourself and never show contempt for yourself in public? Do you deal gently with your imperfections, keep a sense of humor about your foibles, "and with a breath of kindness, blow the rest away"?

You must become an expert in caring for your own precious life. You must finally give to yourself the quality of friendship you have been showering on others.

Today, extend the gentle hand of friendship to the only person who can give you the winning life you desire.

*Today's Action Plan: I will be a loving friend to myself. My friendship will not be based on what my weight is, but on what my need is.*

### January 5            Practicing Confidence

*In quietness and in confidence shall be your strength.*
                            *—Isaiah 30:15*

The second principle of your action plan says, "Practice confidence every day." "How can I be confident," you might ask, "when I'm a failure?" First, you're not a failure, and second, this principle doesn't tell you to *be confident* but to *practice confidence.* There's a difference.

It would be silly to advise anyone to walk out in the world and be confident. But *practicing* confidence is considerably easier to do, and produces the same results. Every day as you read and think about your action plan, you gain skill in the practice of confidence. People will be moved by your belief in yourself and the conviction you display, and they will reflect back to you the confidence they see.

Today, notice how each principle in the action plan relates to the others. Because you developed faith in your unique worth with the first principle, you will begin to radiate confidence with the second.

*Today's Action Plan: I will practice confidence until the act of practice becomes the essential me.*

*You gotta accentuate the positive, eliminate the negative.*

—*Johnny Mercer*

Are you holding back from your weight goal because it might threaten someone? Do you feel being overweight makes you a safer, less competitive friend, relative, mate, or lover? You can't afford that. If you are suppressing your goals for someone else's sake, then somewhere you got the idea that success depends on acceptance by others, even negative people. And if your self-acceptance depends totally on pleasing others, you are setting yourself up for failure.

Are you trying to get everyone to like you, even people who are a negative force in your life? We all love approval, but seeking approval becomes an unhealthy activity if we look for it from people who don't support our living and weight goals.

Today, make a first step toward becoming your own person. Accentuate friendships with positive, supportive people. You are no longer willing to live in the shadow of someone else's ego.

*Today's Action Plan: I will not abandon my action plan to gain approval. I will not be defeated before I have begun to fight.*

*The only power which can resist the power of fear is the power of love.*

—*Alan Paton*

The third principle in your action plan says, "Radiate warmth." Become an expert in caring. We are often so afraid others won't like us that our fear is misinterpreted as icy reserve. How you feel about yourself is what you project to others. If you project warmth and show that you care about yourself (even if you have to make a real effort at first), others will mirror that in their response to you.

By radiating warmth and caring, you are showing the world that you have a reservoir of love, that you have made a positive decision about yourself that you are going to share with others.

Today, understand that each step in your action plan helps you move stride-by-stride down the winning road in life.

*Today's Action Plan: I will discover the changes that warmth and caring will bring into my life. I will overpower my fear with love.*

## January 8 — Don't Ask Yourself the Wrong Questions

*No question is so difficult to answer as that to which the answer is obvious.*

—George Bernard Shaw

"Why can't I do anything right? What's wrong with me?" Some overeaters seem to wallow in destructive self-questioning, hopelessness, self-belittling, and put-downs. Most of the time, these are silent statements that create a continuing negative monologue.

Self-questioning can be positive, if it's done to discover where you went wrong and how to avoid the same mistake in the future. But if you keep on asking, "What's wrong with me?" you'll soon convince yourself that everything you do is wrong, that you will fail. And fail you will.

Send your mind positive questions instead. Ask, "What did I do right?" and "How could I do even better?" You need an inner voice that's a friend, not an enemy, one that's smart, positive, and true.

Today and every day, ask yourself out loud, "What have I done right?" If you ask yourself "right" questions, you will get "right" answers.

*Today's Action Plan: I will ask, "What is good about me?" I will not abuse myself, but be a loving friend.*

## January 9                    The Greatest De-motivator

*The only thing we have to fear is fear itself.*
                              *—Franklin D. Roosevelt*

The fourth principle in your action plan says, "Learn what your fears are." Essentially, most of us are afraid of one thing: failure. We call it by many other names, but behind them all lurks the fear of lost prestige.

It's good to take a daily inventory of your fears because fear—the biggest de-motivator of all—stops you cold. Fear is a habit that has little to do with reality. And we overeaters often turn to food to give us the comfort and security fear takes from us.

From this day on, replace fear with what you desire from life. Think about the healthful thin body you want and let this positive image motivate you.

Today, take the first small step toward ridding your life of its load of fear. You will become a help, not a burden, to yourself.

*Today's Action Plan: I will overcome fear by denying it the power to make me overeat. I will remember that fear is only False Evidence Appearing Real.*

*The future starts today, not tomorrow.*
                                    *—Pope John Paul II*

"I'll think about that tomorrow," said Scarlett O'Hara in the last scene of *Gone With the Wind*. That may be all right for Miss Scarlett in her scheme to get Rhett Butler back, but for the rest of us it's a loser's philosophy.

Don't hedge your commitment to a new life by endless postponing. "I'll start a healthy, lifetime eating program tomorrow," you say, "or Monday, or New Year's Day."

Starting today—right now—commit yourself to diet success. Don't weaken your resolve to do the difficult things you must do with an I'll-give-it-a-try attitude. Don't excuse yourself from an all-out effort.

It's really exciting to know that you will not deny yourself what you want from life. Defying procrastination is one good habit that guarantees success.

Today, commit yourself to a positive new way of thinking about the future. *Today*, not tomorrow, is the beginning of the rest of your life.

*Today's Action Plan: I will replace the bad habit of procrastination with the good habit of working for what I want. I will start from where I am, as I am.*

**January 11**                          **The Good Craving**

*Desire: to wish or long for; crave.*
                              *—American Heritage Dictionary*

The fifth principle in your action plan says, "Acknowledge a burning desire to be thin and healthy."

You need the desire to succeed. Nobody can be a winner without enormous desire, and the more you desire, the more you will help yourself do what it takes to lose weight. Focus on specific goals: a twenty-pound loss, strong legs, a new swimsuit.

We overeaters like to keep our desires secret—even from ourselves. If we don't acknowledge how much we want to be thin, it won't hurt so much if we fail. But our desires power our drive to win. Rather than hide them, we should hold them out in front of us as we develop positive cravings for them.

Today, turn the liability of craving into an asset. You have begun to harness the power of the desire to succeed.

*Today's Action Plan: I will acknowledge to myself and to others my burning desire to be thin and healthy. I will use my craving power to move toward my weight goal.*

## January 12                                  Begin Where You Are

*Don't let life discourage you; everyone who got where he is had to begin where he was.*
*—Richard L. Evans*

You want to lose weight and free the essential you that lives inside a prison of fat, but you're having trouble starting. Even a desperate desire to lose weight doesn't show you how to begin, does it?

Start any way, anywhere, and the pieces will fall into place. When you ask, "How can I get the answer so that I can begin?" the reply comes: "Begin so you can get the answer."

Just as you are, you are complete. You are capable of beginning just where you are.

Today, see that just by starting you are a step closer to achieving. The time and place to begin are right now and right here—and for all you're worth.

*Today's Action Plan: I will believe that the time to start is now. I will begin from wherever I am to find my answer on the other side of action.*

**January 13**                    **You Are Your Sunshine**

*A man should learn to watch that gleam of light which flashes across his mind from within.*
                              *—Ralph Waldo Emerson*

The sixth principle in your action plan says, "Make your own sunlight." Don't wait for everyone else to feel good before you do; take charge of your own happiness.

Why should your happiness depend on other people and events? Why should you be enthusiastic and full of joy only when everybody else is up? That takes the power out of your inner self and places it in the hands of other people.

Being happy is one habit you should cultivate. Work on the happiness habit. Your habits are your choices.

Today, see happiness as a light that shines from the inside out. As with every step in your action plan, if you want it, do it.

*Today's Action Plan: I will light my own way to happiness. I won't wait for others, but will take action myself.*

**January 14**                    **Put Some Style in Your Life**

*Life is a mirror and will reflect back to the thinker what he thinks into it.*
                              *—Ernest Holmes*

*Lifestyle* popularly means a mode of life such as the new one you are creating for yourself with the action plan in this book. But it also implies that your life can have style, your own unique style, which you are developing by committing to a thinner, healthier life and a new love for yourself. In this context, *style* conveys a sense of permanence, not fad; of continuity, not fashion; of an anchor, not something you put on and take off easily.

When you select your healthy eating plan, choose physical exercise, and adopt positive attitudes, these things *become* your lifestyle. They help you build new habits of success and sustain them. You move from self-awareness to action-oriented self-understanding. You acquire the kind of faith and optimism that winners possess—you know you can succeed.

Today, adopt the idea of having a life with style. Great success is on its way.

*Today's Action Plan: I will choose my own lifestyle. I will base it on a vision of victory.*

**January 15**                    **The Most Important Action You Can Take**

*The world is for those who make their dreams come true.*

*—Harold Gray*

You're reading this book because you think it can help you lose weight and maintain that loss. But unlike other "diet" books, this one offers a mental diet that not only ensures weight loss, but guarantees a more satisfying life.

Commit all your energy to the seventh principle in your action plan (the most important of all), which says, "Take charge of your life." If life is a feast, be the host, not the guest.

That doesn't mean that you should belligerently yell, "I'm mad as hell and I'm not going to take it anymore!" That's angry self-pity thinly disguised as action, and it kills everything in you that it takes to be a winner.

Today, you've learned to take the most important action of all. You are ready to take responsibility for yourself and create your own living plan.

*Today's Action Plan: I will take charge of my own life. At the feast of life, I will sit at the head of the table.*

### January 16                                    Yes, You Can

*What goes around, comes around.*
                                        —Contemporary saying

When you're overweight, it's easy to feel depressed, frustrated, humiliated, rejected, deprived, and punished. But winners can't allow such negative feelings to interfere with their goals.

If you catch yourself thinking or saying, "I can't lose ten pounds," reply out loud, "Yes, I can!" You will hear yourself taking charge of your weight problem. And your confident voice will drown out the little voice inside that whispers all too logically: "You've always failed before; you'll fail again."

A diet of negative thinking guarantees you'll fail; nourishing yourself with positive responses guarantees you'll win.

Today, realize that the fight against fat may be as much in your head as on your plate.

*Today's Action Plan: Very few people get to where I want to go, but I can be one who succeeds.*

*Dost thou love life? Then do not squander time; for that's the stuff life is made of.*

*—Benjamin Franklin*

The eighth principle in your action plan says, "Do whatever has to be done *now*." Today, take the action that will change your life.

It's true that stress comes with any diet, job, or social change. But you are stressed much more from changes that are thrust upon you than from your own take-charge changes.

Refusal to change, to grow, and to meet challenges cuts the pattern of defeat deep into your life. Focus not on how often you fail, but on how many times you win. You'll find that you win in direct proportion to the number of times you fail, but keep on beginning again. Get to work on today's task. Beginning again and again is the stuff each day is made of.

*Today's Action Plan: I will get on with my life's work. I will use each minute because it will never come again.*

*Everything has been said before, but since nobody listens we have to keep going back and beginning all over again.*

*—André Gide*

We overweight people are often such people-pleasers. We say *yes* to everyone so they'll like us, maybe even forget we're fat.

But when it comes to pleasing ourselves, we often say *no*. We say *no* to ourselves, to our dreams, and to our desires.

It's time to learn to say yes. Say yes to an eating plan that will help you take off your excess weight and keep it off.

Learn to work positively with yourself. When there is more *yes* than *no* in your life, you will wake each morning to an exciting day that you'll look forward to. Today say yes, and mean it.

*Today's Action Plan: I will take* no *out of my life and put* yes *in.*


**January 19**                                                    **Step by Step**

*If you have no idea where you want to go, it makes little difference how fast you travel.*
                                                    *—Italian proverb*

The ninth principle in your action plan is "Take weight loss in steps." Always aim for a weight goal that excites you, but doesn't frighten you. Then when you reach that goal, start the process all over again until you reach your ultimate goal.

Setting goals is easy for most overeaters. We're such all-or-nothing people that, in the first wave of enthusiasm, we decide to lose all our excess weight *now.* We're fine until problems make us stumble, then depression sets in and we overeat. This is a scene most of us have enacted again and again.

Who created this scene? You did, by setting unrealistic goals. Instead, aim first for an attainable goal. Stop there and say, "Well done." Then start again.

Today, set reasonable priorities, well thought out in advance. You'll be thrilled by achieving your first weight goal.

*Today's Action Plan: I will set my next goal. I will write it down and commit myself to reaching it.*

*Unfortunately, people ask more of car salesmen than they do about new diets. Some of the fads that have been promoted are outrageous.*

—Dr. Peter Wood

Many weight control plans provide a meal-by-meal listing of what to eat for a specified period. With the menus are usually two other lists: one list of foods you can eat in unlimited quantities, another list of foods you should avoid totally. This kind of diet may be one way to get started, but as soon as possible you should choose your own healthy eating plan.

You need a new definition of *diet*. Think of it not as something to "go on" and eventually "go off," but as the way you want to live with food now and forever, an integral part of your lifestyle.

The best diet plan is one that follows general nutritional guidelines, one that calls for a sensible mixture of protein and carbohydrates. Your plan should be high in natural fiber, with plenty of grains, fruits, and vegetables. It should be low in salt, sugar, and fats. Red meats and dairy products, if allowed, should be used in moderation. This is a diet for energy, health, and weight control.

Today, use these guidelines to choose your healthy eating plan.

*Today's Action Plan: I will choose a diet I can live with for a lifetime. I will make it an important part of my lifestyle.*

*If fifty million people say a foolish thing, it is still a foolish thing.*

—Anatole France

The tenth principle in your action plan says, "Reject rejection firmly and totally." How much do you depend on the opinion of others? When your mate or a friend disapproves of your new resolve, what do you do? Do you back off from your goals rather than risk upsetting that person?

If people reject you because they don't like your goals, reject their rejection, completely. What they're really objecting to is your emerging independence; they see you are no longer dependent on their awareness, but are inner-directed toward your own.

You might be lonely for a time; you might even miss looking up to someone for acceptance. But that's a small price to pay for finally being able to take charge of your life.

Today, see how the trap of dependence is built, so you can work your way out of it. You have gladly traded dependence for independence.

*Today's Action Plan: I will reject rejection. I will be a self-directed person.*

## January 22                                    Your Full Life

*Life can be so full, if you use it.*
—*Laura Z. Hobson*

One of the dictionary definitions of the word *use* is "to consume." When applied to life, that's an interesting concept for overeaters. Instead of excess food, life itself is what we should be devouring.

As the contemporary axiom says, we should "use it or lose it." If you don't approach life with zest every day, you can lose it a day at a time.

Plan your time. If you don't know how, start with this simple, effective system: Set aside a few minutes every morning and actually write down the action you're going to concentrate on for the rest of the day, action that is aimed at achieving your weight goal. Plan each day so you can live life to the brim.

Today, use life instead of allowing it to use you. You have found a daily system of using your precious time.

*Today's Action Plan: I will plan my time today. I will make full use of every minute.*

## January 23                          Change—the Challenge

*Risk is essential. There is no growth or inspiration in staying within what is safe and comfortable.*
                                        *—Alex Noble*

The eleventh principle in your action plan says, "Don't fight inevitable change." Changes come in your life, no matter what you do to stop them. And the best changes are those you control. Look back at the changes in your life thus far, those forced on you and those you chose. Which ones made you feel more in charge of your own destiny?

As you reflect on the changes you've experienced, determine which ones added the knowledge you need to march ahead to a healthier, happier, winning life. Your inner self instinctively knows when changes are positive and when they are negative. Looking within will also help you discover the unconscious negative motivations that make you use food in ways you do. And you can use this knowledge, in turn, to make positive change.

Today, accept that change is a part of life's system and that, whenever possible, you will make your own choices.

*Today's Action Plan: I will control change when I can, so that from now on I will be the driver, not the pas-senger.*

*Keep on keeping on.*
                    *—Alcoholics Anonymous saying*

You have hope that you can lose weight, although sometimes that hope seems to be a little flame ready to flicker out. But somehow it doesn't. You go on, because you have courage. That's what hope is, the courage to go on, even in the face of defeat.

Reading this book, thinking about it, and putting its ideas into action illustrates your bravery. You have the courage to live with a food problem in our thin culture, and you keep that tiny pilot light of hope glowing. This book is about *continuing*, the character trait that will lead you to lifelong triumphs.

Today, see that your tiny flame of hope can burst into full blaze with the slightest encouragement.

*Today's Action Plan: I will recognize that my average life is made above average by the hope I keep alive. I will put my courage into action and follow my eating plan.*

*There is always an enormous temptation in all of life to diddle around. . . . it is so self-conscious, so apparently moral, simply to step aside from the gaps where the creeks and winds pour down, saying, I never merited this grace . . . and then sulk along the rest of your days on the edge of rage. I won't have it.*
                    *—Annie Dillard*

The twelfth and last of the principles in your action plan says, "Play life to win." Many people are apathetic about their own welfare. Beyond their immediate desires, they are satisfied just to get by. But you want to achieve more; you want to succeed. You want some peace of mind, a way out of the pit of overeating.

Life's winners don't get to be winners because they "diddle around." They set goals and take action to achieve them. By the time they reach their goals, they have learned to love themselves enough to believe they deserve what they've worked so hard for.

Today, decide that life is too short to wander around with no goal in mind. Believe that you deserve what you get.

*Today's Action Plan: I will not fool around in this life waiting to be rescued. I won't settle for failure!*

## January 26          Work Your Action Plan

*Nothing is impossible to the man who can will, and then do; this is the only law of success.*
        —Honoré Mirabeau

Do more than just read the action plan. Study it, memorize it, let the ideas sink in. In this book, we'll go back to it again and again. It takes a lot of repeating to undo years of overeating.

Expect to have a few rough days. Just don't forget that if you'll keep on working, keep on learning, keep on doing, the rough period will pass and the good days will come.

Don't make losing weight a chore. Schedule nonfood rewards when you've earned them, and don't miss taking them. Rewards help you maintain a strong drive toward your goal.

Give yourself a positive nonfood reward today, like recreation, a new gadget, or anything you really want. Keep your motivation and will to win high; take the rewards you earn.

*Today's Action Plan: I will take one action step at a time, again and again. My life will be beautiful.*

*There is no dependence that can be sure but a dependence on one's self.*
                                                    *—John Gay*

Many weight-control programs you tried may have failed simply because they didn't fit you as an individual. They demanded too many compromises of your lifestyle. The program was master and you were the servant.

No single weight-loss or exercise regimen is exactly right for everybody. There are many good plans, but they are only foundations on which to build your own way of eating and energizing. Learning how to take care of your body and your life is an independent process. No one can hand you a ready-made solution; you must develop the one that works for you.

Discover your own path to physical and mental fitness today. Become the primary expert on your own life.

*Today's Action Plan: I will take responsibility for my own life plan. I will follow my personalized schedule to independence.*

*Let no one or anything stand between you and the difficult task. . . . Do it better each time. Do it better than anyone else can do it. I know this sounds old-fashioned. It is, but it has built the world.*
                                                *—Harlow H. Curtice*

Are you saying, "If I were younger . . .," or, "If I weighed less . . .," or, "If I were smarter, I'd try to work my action plan"? Only *if* stands between you and fulfillment.

Whether you just started a weight-control program or you've been at it for years, determine today that you will make your action plan pay off.

Absorb each day's message in this book. Concentrate while you read. Firmly plant each day's thoughts in your memory. Underline words or phrases that are important to you, or jot them on a slip of paper. Repeat them to yourself during the day. Use what you learn right away to help you live better.

Today, use this book to keep *if* from getting between you and fulfillment.

*Today's Action Plan: I will absorb each day's message. I will use it to help me when* if *gets in my way.*

## January 29                                    The Good Witch

*The Wicked Witch of the West said, "I could make her my slave, for she does not know how to use her power."*
*—L. Frank Baum*

It may seem psychologically easier to blame others for our problems: "That's just another rotten thing my mother did to me," or, "If I had married the right person, I wouldn't need to overeat." We've all looked for someone or something to blame for our extra pounds. But it doesn't get us very far.

Inside you lies the power to do as you want to do, to cooperate with yourself in a new way to eat, to create a new lifestyle. If you don't possess this power over yourself, then who does? Who is responsible for your ability to think, move, and work? Nobody else pulls your strings. You tell yourself to do all of these things, and then you do them.

Today, uncover the good and the powerful in you. Picture yourself as you have always wanted to be: a winner.

*Today's Action Plan: I won't settle for anything less than to learn how to use my own power. When I need strength, I will look to the limitless power of my mind.*

**January 30**                  **Are You Willing?**

*The alcoholic has to be in such pain that he is willing to do anything, even get well!*
           *—Alcoholics Anonymous saying*

Like alcoholism, overeating can be a terrible addiction—with one difference: While the alcoholic can totally abstain from alcohol, the overeater must make a life companion of food.

The overeater's solution is a change in thinking, a change in those ingrained unhealthy food habits. It will take daily vigilance. If you want to overeat, no amount of wishing, willpower, tears, or tantrums can make you give up that inner want.

Yet you certainly don't want the weight gain, health risks, and low self-regard that come with overeating. Can you learn to truly dislike overeating, to hate it?

Today, realize that you are your own jailer. In getting rid of a terrible food addiction, you are not giving up anything good.

*Today's Action Plan: I want to leave overeating behind. I am so sick and tired of pain that I'm willing to get well, no matter what it takes.*

*There are plenty of alibis for failure; success doesn't need them.*

—*Anonymous*

One excitement for every overeater is supreme: the excitement and deep satisfaction of reaching a weight goal and then going on to a new one. You are beginning to understand that knowing what you think and why you think that way isn't enough; you must put this knowledge into action.

You have learned the value of time. If you postpone action today, you lose it. No matter how difficult your problem, no matter how long you've lived with it, you have begun to think about how to be good to yourself today.

Every day you live, every move you make is a step toward a thinner body and a healthier attitude. Start by focusing on your goal each day, and then swing into action.

Today, look back over the month of January. Your life is beginning to change—you are learning more about your own mind than you ever knew before.

*Today's Action Plan: I will put my positive new attitudes into action. I will live today as if it were all there was to life.*

**February 1**                                              **Beginning**

*The beginning is half of every action.*
                                              *—Greek proverb*

To be successful, some overeaters need strong motivation to put each day on a positive path. So each day, they perform a ritual of beginning—an inspirational reading, a supportive telephone call to another overeater, a prayer.

Develop your own ritual to put action in every day. Each morning, seek a balance between what the world demands of you and what you must do for yourself.

What do you want to accomplish today? You can make anything happen—the choice is and has always been yours. To strengthen that belief, exercise your positive mental attitude; the more you exercise it, the stronger it becomes.

Today, develop a positive ritual for starting each day. You are taking charge; you are setting goals.

*Today's Action Plan: I will make a good beginning. I will exercise my positive mental muscles.*

**February 2**                                          **Establish Routine**

*You will never be the person you can be if pressure, tension, and discipline are taken out of your life.*
                                              *—Dr. James G. Bilkey*

Overeaters often lack discipline. Continuous snacking and overemphasis on food can interrupt daily life and make it difficult to maintain schedules.

Setting a time for doing tasks you want to accomplish is beneficial. Repeating an activity at the same time every day helps to make the activity—exercise, for example—habitual.

Prioritize your daily activities. Meal planning for healthy eating should be near the top of your list. Other high priorities are exercise, your daily action plan, and your work and family. All other activities come later.

Set time and priorities for the things you want to accomplish today. Now that you have a plan, you will follow it.

*Today's Action Plan: I will put my new lifestyle priorities first. I will create routines of healthy, happy new habits.*

**February 3**                                    **Are You a List-Maker?**

*Any plan that depends upon luck to succeed isn't a plan; it's a gamble.*

*—Anonymous*

Don't just read this book, use it! When you read an interesting action idea, write it down. List it with the tasks you want to accomplish today. Don't rely on memory or luck to remind yourself to do it.

Make a list of what you want to do today, and then, more important, *do* the tasks. Making the list is not action. *Doing* is the key to your new thin life.

When you have the list habit, you feel more dynamic and goal-oriented. You won't have to waste time wondering what it was you wanted to do with your day, and you'll see progress toward your goals as well.

Today, make a list to help you organize your day and forestall overeating from frustration.

*Today's Action Plan: I will list the activities I want to accomplish. I will organize my day to exclude overeating.*

## February 4                    Is Overeating a Disease?

*Disease: to interrupt or impair any or all the natural and regular functions of an organ of a living body.*
                    —Webster's Unabridged Dictionary

Does habitual overeating impair the regular or natural functions of your body in any way? Have you ever felt hungover, tired, dizzy, or generally debilitated from too much food?

Overeating is a disease of living, and its symptom is fat. Food has become a drug that protects you from a negative personal view of life in which you see yourself always failing, always at the mercy of people and situations.

The disease of excess hunger is curable. You simply have to form a winning view of the world and your place in it. An action plan, healthy eating, and body-rebuilding exercise are the answers.

Today, take steps to cure your overeating disease. Following your action plan is the place to begin.

*Today's Action Plan: Through attitude, proper eating, and exercise, I can recover from my "disease." I will take the prescription of action.*

## February 5                    Oh, What Good Confusion

*Oxymoron: a paradoxical conjunction of terms.*
                    —American Heritage Dictionary

When you seek self-understanding, your mind may indulge in confusion to protect itself from change. If you feel confused, simply accept it as another step toward self-understanding.

Confusion reflects the conflict between what your outer self denies and what your inner self knows. Gradually, as you grow in self-understanding, you will "pull yourself inside out." Don't expect it to come easily. It's a rebirthing process; but during it, you will be unchaining the real, more powerful you.

Today, realize that confusion is part of your learning process. You have caught a glimpse of the fabulous reality within you.

*Today's Action Plan: Step by step, I will gain understanding. I will cultivate an inquiring attitude so I can release my confident inner self.*

### February 6                    Where the Answer Lies

*Be a lamp unto your own feet, do not seek outside yourself.*

*—Buddha*

You might be asking, "What's all this about my inner self? Is this a diet book or isn't it?"

You won't find diets in these pages. You know what you have to eat to reach your target weight. Which diet to follow is not your problem.

*You have to learn to love your self enough to save your self.* That's the answer, and always has been.

It lies within your reach; the cure is in you. But when you cannot face everyday problems, you lose confidence and look around for an escape. An overeater's unhappy escape is lurking behind the refrigerator door.

Your everyday frustrations will usually heal themselves

if you do not overeat. It is that simple. You escape from the fat trap as you seek solutions from within rather than from outside yourself.

Today, ask questions. Where do the answers lie? In self-understanding.

*Today's Action Plan: I will choose one good diet plan and follow it. I will light the lamp of self-understanding.*

### February 7                                            The Other Answer

*When faced with a problem...chances are the solution lies not in a new idea but in a new look at an old one.*
*—George Sheehan*

To achieve the body you want, you must add a physical companion to your diet solution—exercise. Limiting food intake without adding exercise lowers the body's metabolism and eventually makes dieting counterproductive. In other words, the old yo-yo syndrome—losing weight, only to bounce back to a higher weight—is caused not just by overeating, but also by a low-energy life.

The only way you can control your weight permanently is to eat a healthful diet and exercise regularly. And the road to this high-energy living, the lifestyle of a winner, is paved with the bricks of self-understanding. See how it all comes together?

Today, add exercise to your diet. It's the only way to raise your metabolism and stop the weight yo-yo.

*Today's Action Plan: I will do what has to be done now. I will exercise.*

## February 8 — The High-Energy Life

*Nothing is too good to be true.*

*—Ernest Holmes*

To develop a good habit, we must look to ourselves while our feet move toward what we want. No one deprives us of a thinner, healthier body but ourselves. Make it a habit to try new things, to work for what you want.

Do you say: "I am ashamed of myself. I don't deserve anything better. I don't believe there is anything better for me in this world"? Nonsense!

Nothing is too good to be true. The best life you have ever dreamed of is not as good as the truth. Your imagination can conceive of only a fragment of what good can come to you. The thought that you can never have the high-energy life you want is just an old lie. Reach for the best life you can conceive.

Today, put down the lie that you don't deserve better. You have seen that your desires can never exceed your abilities.

*Today's Action Plan: I will get rid of the old lies. I will believe that every good I can imagine can be true.*

## February 9 — Why Self-Esteem Is So Important

*He who finds himself, loses his misery.*

*—Matthew Arnold*

Doing what we know needs to be done is the greatest builder of self-esteem. People who have achieved their desires are achieving what they think they deserve; people who achieve nothing are doing the same thing.

Many people love you. They would give you the self-esteem you need if they could. But the will to achieve doesn't come from the outside; it isn't handed to you or forced on you. The drive to win must come from within you.

Today, find in yourself the will and drive to win. Self-esteem is what powers your desire to win, and self-esteem builds as you do what you must do. This is the magic you've been waiting for.

*Today's Action Plan: I will take charge of building my own self-esteem. From this minute on, I will consider myself a winner.*

### February 10                    Perpetual Motion Engine

*If you would hit the mark, you must aim a little above it.*

—*Henry Wadsworth Longfellow*

Achievement is the greatest motivator. Like a wonderful perpetual motion device, achievement continuously powers you to dare more, go higher, gain further success.

But many of us have excuses for not achieving. We call ourselves late bloomers, slow learners, and, most of all, we have this awful handicap of being overweight.

If you want a healthy, thinner body and a release from a horrible dependency on food, you must make the required investment. Once you invest in yourself, it's not all uphill anymore; just getting into action smoothes the road ahead.

Decide that achievement is worth investing in today. You'll find that you can hit the mark if you give up cherished excuses from the past. Today, you are an achiever.

*Today's Action Plan: I will fly as high as I want to. I will achieve one goal that I have been postponing.*

*Oftentimes nothing profits more than self-esteem, grounded on what is just and right.*

—*John Milton*

How many times has someone made a cruel or insensitive remark about your size? If you think of yourself only as a weight, if you consider yourself an unworthy person, you may believe you deserve this unpardonable attack. How many times have you taken insults because you thought your weight had stripped you of the right to common courtesy?

You may have ignored the person and gone home feeling angry and depressed. But if you had had a healthy sense of self-respect and a sense of inviolable worth, you could have turned and said, "That was a rude remark."

Today you have a new, self-respecting lifestyle. Today, respond firmly to unmannerly remarks or gratuitous advice, or refuse to dignify them with notice.

*Today's Action Plan: I will be self-respectful. I will insist that others—even strangers—treat me with respect.*

**February 12**                    **Three Parts to a Whole**

*You have to go as far as you can see…to see how far you can go.*

—*Anonymous*

You have resolved to turn your life around 180 degrees so your future will be unburdened by overeating problems. At this point, your new lifestyle must contain a powerful threesome: a weight-losing food program, a physical fitness program, and a mental fitness program. It is essential that you adopt all three parts of your new action program at once.

Sustained overeating and the resultant bouts of grief, frustration, and panic once impaired your physical and mental systems. But now you have a positive new three-part cure. Healthful eating, an energized body, and positive, creative attitudes together produce healing through real physical and biochemical changes.

Today, become engrossed in a three-part positive plan for weight loss, physical fitness, and mental fitness. You have everything you need.

*Today's Action Plan: I will write all three parts of my new plan on paper. I will commit myself to wellness.*

## February 13                    Watch Out for Self-Criticism

*By despising himself too much a man comes to be worthy of his own contempt.*
*—Henri-Frédéric Amiel*

A popular pastime for many overweight people is to participate in sprees of self-criticism. Perhaps you have berated yourself publicly to show how psychologically sensitive and knowledgeable you are. This is a wrong-headed way of gaining approval. No matter how sincere, it has a negative impact on your self-image.

If our thoughts alone can help us visualize ourselves, then how much more do our spoken words influence others' and our own opinions of us? Have you ever complained about yourself to a companion, saying, for instance, "I'm always so afraid in groups," only to have your friend parrot back to you later, "Oh, you can't do that, you're afraid in groups." Your spoken negative image judged you in another's mind and was reinforced by your friend's words.

Today, learn to speak positively about yourself. Your own words can be powerful weapons.

*Today's Action Plan: I will not play the self-criticism game. I will reinforce the positive and powerful in me, out loud.*

## February 14                                    One Way Out

*Admitting a problem is halfway to solution.*

*—Anonymous*

Are you having trouble admitting that you have a weight problem? Are you still talking about baby fat, a big frame, and glands? Until you admit that you are an overeater, you can't begin to whip your weight problem. *The way to get out of trouble is to first realize you're in trouble.*

If you don't see your pounds as your problem to solve, you probably see yourself as a victim of fate. Victims gain nothing but pounds and pity. When overeaters can't admit their problem and take charge of the solution, the world leaves them behind. You, and you alone, can make life work for you.

Today, admit you have a problem with food, then start working on a solution.

*Today's Action Plan: I admit that I have an eating problem. I will follow a program of self-understanding, eating, and exercise that will make my life work beautifully.*

## February 15                                         Feelings

*Feelings are not reasons.*

*—Alfred Adler*

Do you use your feelings as an excuse to do what you know you should not? When you are disappointed, hurt, or angry, do you say, "I feel so bad, I can't help

eating"? To be ruled by such feelings makes you a helpless victim of emotion.

It's the old pain of self-pity again. Remembered hurts
never die—they lurk in your mind, ready to rationalize
destructive habits. They become reasons.

Feelings, used as reasons, are alibis for not taking
charge of your life. You'll function best if you keep a
certain emotional distance between what happens to
you and your reaction to it.

Today, recognize the positive difference between reasons and feelings.

*Today's Action Plan: No matter how bad I feel, I will
not return to overeating. I will not allow self-pity to
rule my emotions.*

**February 16**                                **New Habit for Old**

*Forming a new habit is like winding string on a ball.*
                                              *—William James*

Losing weight means forming a new habit of healthy
eating, a continuing process. Give it time. The longer
you wind the string philosopher William James talked
about, the further ahead you'll be. If you drop the
string, pick it up and begin to wind again. The stronger
a new habit gets, the less compelling the temptation is
to drop the ball.

When you form the new habit of healthy eating and
attain that thinner body you want, the rewards are fantastic. You see your worth because you are beginning to
understand more about yourself.

What is your next weight goal? Write it down.
Writing is action, and every day you are putting action
into your life.

Today, make a new habit happen. Decide to "wind

string" until your new habit of healthy eating becomes stronger than the old habit of overeating.

*Today's Action Plan: I will make a good new habit stronger every day. I will follow my action plan as a doer, not a regretter.*

### February 17                  For Me—Right Now!

*If I am not for myself, who is for me? And when I am for myself, what am I? And if not now, when?*
> *—Hillel*

It's too late for you to go back to your self-destructive ways. By now, you have learned a new way of thinking and have gained the self-understanding that compels you to go forward.

The past is buried; today you are beginning your future. This minute should be one of the happiest of your life because you are getting rid of the compulsion to use food destructively.

The more you understand, the harder it will be for you to turn around and go back to the negative rationalizations you once made; all the tired excuses just won't work anymore. Self-knowledge has detoured any overeating pleasure you once might have had.

Today, follow the road ahead to achievement. It really is easier than the road back to overeating.

*Today's Action Plan: I will walk on. I will enjoy this day because I am for me, right now.*

### February 18        Don't Use This Book as an Excuse

*If you don't want to do something, one excuse is as good as another.*
> *—Yiddish saying*

Some overweight people have found help from a weight-losing group, a doctor, a spa, or a spiritual adviser. Outside support systems are very helpful, but it's still important to use your action plan and read this book. The key to every weight-loss or maintenance program is motivation, and it's difficult for any overeater to get enough motivation on a day-to-day basis. The group may not be meeting, the doctor or spiritual adviser is on vacation, or the spa is closed. That's what this book gives you, a friend at hand every time you need a boost.

As for the other helpful techniques you've allowed into your weight-loss program, who do you think made the decision to let them in and let them stay? That's one of the greatest take-charge decisions of all.

There are many ways you can help yourself, and you're doing one of them today: You are reading this book and getting into action.

*Today's Action Plan: I will take all the help I can get. I will add action to whatever other help I have in my life.*

**February 19**                              **Who We Are**

*Character is a victory, not a gift.*

*—Anonymous*

Action is character; we are what we do. We can talk about what we will do someday, but unless what we say agrees with our action, it is meaningless.

In a way, idle talk and addiction are much the same. They are both means of avoiding action. You might say, "That's unfair, I really do have big plans. I'm just waiting for the right time to come along." Of course you try to believe it, to cushion the pain of living a low-energy, nonachieving life. But have you fooled yourself with this alibi?

What you do is what you truly mean. There is only one way to live—in direct contact with today.

To be a winner, you must act, today. You, and you alone, can change your life.

*Today's Action Plan: I will not be caught in the trap of talking instead of doing. I will follow the eighth principle of my action plan and do whatever has to be done now.*

**February 20**                    **Are You Rolling a Rock Uphill?**

*Every time you act, you add strength to the motivating idea behind what you've done.*

*—George Weinberg*

In Greek mythology, Sisyphus was a king condemned by Zeus to roll a stone to the top of a hill. All day, he rolled it toward the top, but when he stopped at night, the stone rolled to the bottom of the hill again. Sisyphus was doomed to roll his stone up the hill every day.

Overeating is like the burden of the Sisyphus stone. A new life, one that pulls you away from your no-win dependence, won't come easily. But there's loveliness and beauty in living free of your compulsion.

Soon positive new habits will overwhelm your negative old habits. Once this happens, your Sisyphus stone will stay at the top of your mountain. Persistence is the key.

Today, commit yourself to a healthful winner's life. Whatever it takes, you know you will provide yourself with the desire to succeed.

*Today's Action Plan: I will win and be thin. By eating right one day at a time, I will stay on top of the mountain forever.*

*It is impossible to underrate human intelligence.*
                                            —*Henry Adams*

The ideas embodied in the principles of your action plan are for you. They were designed to lift you up, to open your mind to all the possibilities that you have buried for so long behind a barrier of flesh.

Today, you are another person. Some part of you is born anew today and will be born anew tomorrow. Your yesterdays have no power over you unless you allow them the power.

What was true a few months ago was true for a different person. Today you are developing the unique human being that you are. Your confidence is growing. You have a desire to succeed, and you want to get into action.

Today, refuse to allow yesterday's failure to punish the winning new person you have become. Give yourself a fresh new start every day.

*Today's Action Plan: I will use my action plan as a way to a higher understanding of myself. I will give this new me every possible chance.*

*To err is human, to forgive divine.*
                                            —*Alexander Pope*

In this often-quoted line, you probably think Pope was talking about forgiving other people, and perhaps he was. But there is another forgiveness that you haven't practiced: self-forgiveness.

Self-hate causes you to condemn yourself. You say, "I'll never be able to stick to this diet," and then you make your prediction come true.

The only way out of your own trap is to *forgive yourself!* You can't live a high-energy, action-oriented, achieving life until you practice self-forgiveness. It's the foundation for a life that knows more joy than pain, more success than failure. And you must forgive yourself again and again.

Today, deny that failure image, and accept the intelligent, lovable, winning you. You must give yourself a chance before you can give anything to anyone else.

*Today's Action Plan: I will find a new love. It will be me.*

## February 23                    Have the Time of Your Life

*Time is no speedway between the cradle and the grave but space to find a place in the sun.*
                                        —*Phil Bosmans*

It's never going to be today again; that's the essence of the eighth principle in your action plan. That means you should live in the present and not waste a moment. It does not mean you shouldn't plan for the future, just don't worry about it. Planning is action, whereas worrying is a passive victim's game.

Only when you want to live every moment as fully and as serenely as possible will you have the courage to change and the wisdom to believe you can. Learn to love knowledge and change, and time will not drag, but race along. Give yourself some time to laugh and to dance. You have earned it.

Your time is so full of positive activities that you know you are alive. Today, see that you can do astonishing, unique things with the minutes and hours of your day.

*Today's Action Plan: I will not kill time. I will take the gift of time and use it.*

**February 24**                    **The Pain in Gain Is**
                                   **Mainly in the Brain**

*People will say the pain was all in my mind, which is true. But that's the worst place to have it.*
                                        *—Maury Wills*

When you get up enough courage to get on the scale after a weight gain, you're not hurting anywhere but in your self-esteem. Those hated new pounds mean you've cheated yourself. Why don't you do what you know you must do?

You don't because your push is in conflict with your shove; you push forward your desire to be thin and your anxieties shove back—hard. The result of that pain is weight gain.

But you can face that pain! Perhaps you've avoided pain before, maybe with an extra snack or two. Feel it this time, because that pain can teach. How much pain do you need before you've had enough? Are you ready to look at life beyond excess food? Your pain has taught you that you are.

Today, realize that once you are willing to experience and take the responsibility for the pain of overeating, you are ready to push forward to the body you most desire.

*Today's Action Plan: I will accept my pain and understand its lesson. I will practice pushing my desire for a healthy new body past my anxieties.*

*[When you were young] you were always full of the future: some day you are going to do this. And some day is here or it's never going to be here. It's frightening, as if a needle got stuck in the record of life.*
                                                                            *—Cynthia Ozick*

No matter what your age, today is vital. In this hectic world, there are so many demands on your time you must set priorities. Overeaters often put themselves at the bottom of their priority list. Do you do this?

Always make time for the things you want for you. How many times have you promised yourself, "When I have more time, I'll start a good diet and exercise program"?

You will never have more time than you do today. You may think you are too busy to pay attention to your eating problem, but you spend more time agonizing, rationalizing, and self-pitying than you admit. The more time you devote to your own needs, the more you'll be able to accomplish for yourself and others.

Today, examine ways you lose precious time, time you can't afford to waste. Decide that today is that once far-off "someday."

*Today's Action Plan: I will use all the time I have for accomplishment. I will not wait for "someday." I'll pay attention to me now.*

*The cause of obesity could be almost anything.*
                                                                        *—Dr. Albert Stunkard*

Being overweight is complex. Some people become overweight as children, others as adults. Some people eat too much; others burn calories too slowly. Over-weight people come in every size, with mild, moderate, and severe weight problems.

What's the cause? It could be hormones, genes, personality, or a world of convenience that makes food readily available to inactive people. It could be any combination of factors. It doesn't seem fair.

But just because you may be *predisposed* to be over-weight doesn't mean you have to *be* overweight. Try these remedies: right-eating for your individual body, exercise to improve your fat-converting capacity, and positive action. You need to live a richer life now.

Today, face your overweight problem, no matter how unfair it seems, and take charge.

*Today's Action Plan: I will live fully right now, building a new lifestyle that works. I won't worry about what's fair; instead, I'll concentrate on what's necessary.*

## February 27                How Winners Take Rejection

*What lies behind us and what lies before us are tiny matters compared with what lies within us.*
*—William Morrow*

How do you take rejection? Do you feel as if you have been personally attacked? Do you slink away to nurse your wounds and then binge to get even? After your binge, does your anger turn to self-loathing?

This is why the first principle in your action plan is so important. If you know your unique worth, you can handle rejection or criticism without hiding behind excess food.

Winners fight rejection by trying again and again. They solve the problem if they can; then they forget it and walk on. With this attitude, *you may be rejected but you cannot be defeated.*

Don't let others destroy your happiness and don't cooperate with them if they try. Most of the time, they're merely rejecting an idea, an invitation, or an offer, not you.

Today, find a positive side to rejection; see it as an opportunity to change others' ideas about you. Go ahead, show them!

*Today's Action Plan: I will not take rejection personally. I will accept my unique worth so that rejection will simply seem like another challenge, another way to win.*

**February 28**                    **Which Is to Be Master?**

*"The question is," said Humpty Dumpty, "which is to be master—that's all."*

*Lewis Carroll*

Without purpose in our lives, we wallow in self-pity, trying desperately to find a way out of an eating problem we can't control.

We become ready to give up anything but food. We said, "I'd give my right arm if I could only be thin." We pray, cry, and are humbled by others. We see that our lives are becoming more and more unmanageable because of our obsession. Finally, we admit that in order to get some sanity into our eating habits, we have to follow a new and disciplined way of eating.

When you accept a new way of eating, you have purpose in your life—you are the master of your life. By bringing order into your eating, you see that you can have the strength to make changes. Most of all, you discover the force of positive thinking, positive feeling, and positive doing. You can discover who you really are.

Today, see that you are the master of your life. Recognize your obligation to give yourself the best life you can.

*Today's Action Plan: I will accept mastery over my life. I have discovered the power of positive thinking, feeling, and doing.*

**February 29**                                    **Born Again**

*Bare winter suddenly was changed to spring.*
                                        —*Percy Bysshe Shelley*

Are you ready for your rebirth? Are you ready to relinquish the negative patterns of thinking and living which have resulted in a dreary winter of living?

Take a positive idea such as I am *alive, alert, and enthusiastic.* Become this idea. Get inside it; pull it around you like a light spring coat. Make it live.

If spring's rebirth is a universal natural force, why not use this positive force to become the person you want to be. If you do not have a program of eating which will ensure health and weight loss, get one today. If you do not possess the positive attitudes you need to build a growth-centered life, develop them today.

*Today's Action Plan: I will deal with unhappy feelings without eating over them. I will spring into action.*

## March 1                                   Lost and Found

*I have been all my life in hiding.*

—*Kate Millett*

When you take charge of your eating and your life, it's like being found—but even more, it's like coming out of hiding. When we hide from ourselves, we don't know ourselves. There is no greater loneliness. In trying to find comfort, we became dependent on food and found only misery. We became lost.

But things are different now. Every day you are finding your way back to life. You have come out of hiding. You know you can climb out of the pit of loneliness, using your action plan to gain self-understanding.

It is hard to believe it could be that simple. But when you come out of hiding and take charge of your life, your loneliness will disappear and along with it your addiction to overeating.

Today, decide never to hide from yourself again. Your healthy eating and exercise plan for a winning life is your statement of belief in yourself.

*Today's Action Plan: I will believe in my ability to win. I will never hide again.*

*The only way to make me feel better was to make everyone else feel worse.*

> —*Diet group member*

Compulsive overeaters often harbor an unconscious wish for revenge, an indirectly expressed aggression born of anger and resentment against others, but mostly against themselves.

We appear to be vindictive with others—family, friends, co-workers—but our behavior is really just another way of getting even with ourselves for the awful way we feel about overeating. We become our own worst punishers.

No one needs to be punished, least of all you. Forget about getting even. Instead, get thinner, healthier, more successful. How you feel about what you do will determine how you feel about yourself.

Today, replace the silent scream of anger with constructive action. It is far more rewarding to reach out for the good life than to punish yourself for the past.

*Today's Action Plan: I will avoid angry conflict. I will feel only positive things about myself.*

**March 3**                               **How to Avoid Success**

*Tall trees take a lot of wind.*

> —*Flemish saying*

Here's a surefire method to avoid success: never attempt anything. Never make an action plan; never try to take charge of your life. You can avoid success forever just by never trying. This is the way we protect ourselves from failure.

Are you hiding from possible failures? Are you afraid

to grow tall because you might not be able to "take the wind"? You won't always succeed on the first try; be prepared for that. You are trying to do a very tough thing: give up extra food and get rid of negative behavior. It's difficult, but, yes, you can win.

Today, don't avoid failure, because avoiding it means never giving yourself the chance to win. Though your hunger may be powerful, your desire for a new take-charge way of living is even stronger.

*Today's Action Plan: I will stand tall and take a chance. I will keep trying until I succeed.*

### March 4                                              Changing

*If you're never scared or embarrassed or hurt, it means you never take any chances.*

*—Julia Sorel*

Change means that part of your comfortable old self must die to give birth to your new winning self. Sometimes we can't just relax and let the needed change take over; we fight to keep our familiar overeating ways. But we overeaters—when faced with the visual, emotional, and spiritual results of our overeating—know that we must change.

The eleventh principle in your action plan teaches, "Don't fight inevitable change." Instead make change work for you by facing life's problems honestly and working your way through the emotional thickets. Keep the best of yourself. Then get rid of your negative, destructive habits.

Strength of will leads to accomplishments, and your own strength of will is made up of many strengths, including your faith in a Higher Power and the support of friends and professional advisers. From whatever sources you have constructed your strength of will, you demonstrate it when you decide to take charge of your life.

Today, be determined to face your fear of change so you can make change work for you.

*Today's Action Plan: I will begin to make whatever changes are necessary in my life. I have the strength and the will to do it.*

### March 5                          Be Environment Conscious

*Food is the cheapest and most abundant mood-altering drug on the market.*
                                        —*Anne Scott Beller*

Foods—especially our binge foods—are all around us: on television, menus, and magazines. It's impossible to get rid of this temptation completely, but you can take steps to minimize its influence: if you don't want to eat it, don't have it available.

Be honest about the environment you create. Don't kid yourself that you buy your binge food for your children, your mate, or your guests. When you stock up on binge foods, you're creating a negative environment.

If you don't want to slip, avoid slippery places. Don't turn your own kitchen into the food equivalent of a crack house. It's like living with a clanging fire alarm; there's no serenity.

Achievers structure a safe dieting environment by avoiding binge foods. Today, make your home a safe place to live, grow, and change.

*Today's Action Plan: I will binge-proof my environment. I will stay away from slippery places.*

*God gave us memories so that we might have roses in December.*

                                        —*Sir James M. Barrie*

Overweight people store some of the worst memories: cruel rejections, body embarrassments, lost jobs, chances never taken or never offered. You, too, are filled with such negative memories.

Your memory holds the accumulated knowledge of your past. What you can do today is take charge of your *future* memories. If a memory you have is pleasant, cherish it; if it's painful, throw it out.

Every day you make memories. Funnel today's experiences into tomorrow's happy reflections. If you are committed to a healthy winning life, you have also put yourself in charge of your memories so that they will be a resource in your tomorrows. Make confident, committed, winning memories.

Today, put yourself in control of your future memories. Start building them now.

*Today's Action Plan: I will let go of negative memories. For the future, I will begin to make positive memories.*

*"My people," my soul cried. "Who are my people?"*
                                    —*Rosa Zagnoni Marinoni*

If you feel the need to share your recovery process with other overeaters, consider joining a weight-loss support group.

There's a practical reason for you to join a group: they work. People in groups tend to have higher recovery rates than lone dieters because they have a supportive, accepting environment. The other group members help you learn about yourself and your weight problem. They help you focus your energy, and they show you it is possible to win.

Although overeating may have led you to isolate yourself from others, you'll find yourself looking forward to meetings—to stimulation, knowledge, and camaraderie. You can get more help from strangers who overeat than from others close to you who can't understand why you use food as you do.

Today, give a group of fellow overeaters a chance. The "buddy system" could provide the support you need.

*Today's Action Plan: I will attend a group meeting. I will seek and accept help for my overeating problem.*

## March 8               Gifts

*Those gifts are ever the most acceptable which the giver has made precious.*

*—Ovid*

Are you good to yourself? Do you show yourself love in little ways: a gentle word, a walk in the leaves, a small nonfood gift? Do you find a closer contact with your Higher Power? Do you criticize yourself little, encourage much, and forgive quickly?

To be a whole person, you can't separate your spiritual self from your physical body, for it's within your body that your unique spirit lives. All of this is deeply significant for the winner you are.

Give a gift of yourself to someone else, some other overeater who needs your special understanding. Donate some of your time and energy to your family, neighborhood, or community, beyond yourself and your desires. Nothing builds a sense of personal worth like doing something to make others glad that you were there.

Today, don't neglect your spiritual self. You can endure anything as long as your unconquerable spirit is nourished.

*Today's Action Plan: I will nurture my spirit. I will nurture others through service until my spirit glows.*

**March 9**                    **Are You a "Never-Enougher"?**

*It is curious what shifts we make to escape thinking.*
                            *—Herman Melville*

Some overeaters never get enough—not just of food, but of life. Nothing, no matter what quantity or quality, is ever enough. They always have a feeling of deprivation.

People who feel deprived need to become self-nurturers. They need more self-acceptance and less self-criticism, and they need to accept emotional support and comfort from others. Too often, never-enoughers not only don't care about themselves, but they won't allow others to get close enough to care.

Deliberately choose friends who are affectionate by nature. These are important people to you because they meet your need to feel connected to others emotionally. They help you to feel not only loved, but lovable.

Today, discard the feeling that there is never enough for you. Accept nurturing from yourself and others to replace false feelings of deprivation.

*Today's Action Plan: I will not be a "never-enougher."*
*I will reach out for the emotional support I need.*

*I can promise you that you'll begin to enjoy your work-out.*

—*Dr. Kenneth H. Cooper*

Overweight people who begin an exercise program face problems that never concern thin people. Just the thought of appearing in leotards has probably stopped more overweight people from exercising than any other reason. Bluntly put, exercise can be a source of embarrassment for overweight people.

But embarrassment isn't an adequate excuse for not working toward a high-energy body. Be ingenious. Don't squeeze into uncomfortable workout clothes, hear someone laugh at you, and give up fitness—all in one morning. You've got two better choices: ignore insensitive people and head for the gym, or start your exercise program at home. Then when you begin to firm up your body, you'll have enough exercise success to overrun any vestiges of embarrassment. Have a little exercise success today and you'll have more tomorrow.

Today, decide that nothing will keep you from the high-energy, winning life that you deserve.

*Today's Action Plan: I will not let anything stop me from achieving fitness. Today, I will exercise my body.*

*Don't look back. Something might be gaining on you.*
—*Satchel Paige*

Looking back might mean you haven't defined your next goal. Unclear goals can make you feel wary, as if you're being followed by an unidentified pursuer. It's really the old negative you, scared and calling out,

"You're taking a chance going forward. Wait for me!"

Clearly define your goals along the way. Think of each goal as a hand reaching to pull you forward. Plan to achieve each one—whether it's joining a weight-losing group, asking for a doctor's help, or helping yourself toward physical fitness.

Don't look back unless that's the path you want to take. Don't listen to nay-saying voices. You know where you want to go—forward.

Only through planning and persistence can you make dreams come true. Today, reaffirm the action plan that tells you to aim for achievable weight goals.

*Today's Action Plan: I will look ahead on the path to achievement. I will make a goal and aim straight for it.*

## March 12                    Work, Success, and Exercise

*The high tension and low activity of modern life make a deadly mixture.*

*—Dr. Kenneth H. Cooper*

There is ample frustration in being overweight in a thin-is-best world. But couple it with a high-tension job and you see how an overweight person can be in emotional trouble. Then add debilitating inactivity fostered by our electronic culture. Tension and physical inactivity are your powerful foes.

Exercise leads to a fit body and emotional well-being, but did you know that exercise can also help you deal with your job?

Recent research, compiled by the Illinois Council on Health and Physical Fitness, reveals that job absenteeism drops by 60 percent among people who are actively involved in an exercise program. Exercisers score 70 percent higher in decision-making skills, and 60 percent of them enjoy their work more than the nonexercisers do.

Some companies even give incentives to get their employees exercising. Don't you think you ought to put your energy where the smart money is going?

Today, exercise not just for success in your job, but for your life.

*Today's Action Plan: I will reduce tension in my life with exercise. I will make a career exercise investment.*

## March 13                                      Curiosity

*Try to be one of the people on whom nothing is lost.*
—Henry James

Winners are curious about life: the ordinary as well as the extraordinary, the inner as well as the outer world. The more winners know, the more options they have, and the fuller and richer their lives can be.

But knowledge is only the beginning. To accomplish great things you must also be ready to act on what you know. Knowledge is the foundation, and action is the castle you can build upon it.

Learn good nutrition. Learn about exercise. Learn to seek a sense of wellness. Every day you gain more knowledge, you gain more power to attain your dream.

Today, see that new ideas encourage decisions, inform actions, and discourage self-deception. Knowledge opens the world, so you can choose from so many more options.

*Today's Action Plan: I will absorb knowledge like a sponge. I will put this knowledge into action and win.*

*Grief may be joy misunderstood.*
—*Elizabeth Barrett Browning*

Overweight people may go through two different grief processes. When we're covered with excess flesh, we grieve for the person and body we want to be. The longer we've been overweight the more we feel this grief. After weight loss there's another kind of grief mingled with fear and sadness at the loss of a part of one's self. We lose our sense of identity and get confused. The newly thin person reaches back for that familiar self and sometimes gains weight again.

But you can counter this destructive weight-loss grief experience by redefining yourself as your weight goes down. Working your action plan is part of the redefinition process. Think and act like the person you want to be now so you'll be ready for the new you that begins to emerge.

Today, know that if you "get rid of" your extra weight instead of "losing" it, you will head off any misplaced grief when your new body appears.

*Today's Action Plan: I will get rid of my weight. I will understand that any grief I feel is misunderstood joy.*

*When the horse is dead, get off.*
—*Kirk M. Sorensen*

You have been losing weight regularly and you feel great. You are following your healthy eating plan, exercising, building your winning attitude. You're doing everything you've done right all along, but suddenly your efforts don't show in pounds lost. You've hit a plateau. What now? Too often in the past, the answer has been to recede into self-pity and say, "Forget it! I might as well eat!"

*If you're stuck, change something.* It doesn't matter what—adjust your diet or add a new exercise—the important thing is to take charge. Act on your determination and desire to reach your goal. There is no failure but quitting. Winners never quit, and you're a winner.

Today, you can win despite setbacks if you act on what you know. You can make it happen by planning, persistence, and determination.

*Today's Action Plan: If I am stuck, I will change something. I will always be capable of bettering my past record.*

## March 16                                                    Fear

*Fear of becoming a has-been keeps some people from becoming anything.*
                                                        —*Eric Hoffer*

Are you a worry machine? If so, probably half your fears begin with the words *what if.* With these words, you turn opportunity into difficulty.

When you're afraid that something might happen, you must make plans to deal with that worst possible scenario. Outline all the steps to prevent that scenario from happening, to fix it if it does happen, or to live with it if you can't fix it.

Notice that while you were problem solving, you shut off the worry machine. Now that you've learned how to do that, you can walk on to a more positive attitude. Plan, anticipate, and work toward your future instead of worrying about it.

Today, take charge of your worst possible "what if" so it has no power to haunt you.

*Today's Action Plan: I will turn off my worry machine. No matter what I fear, I will deal with it instead of eating over it.*

## March 17                                One Way to Achieve

*If you want to change what other people think of you, you must change what you think of yourself.*
*—George Bernard Shaw*

Are you trying to get everyone to like you? If so, you are basing your self-acceptance on others' opinions. It's fun to be popular, but it's not necessary for self-esteem. Self-acceptance can't be given to you; it is built from within.

If you seek approval from someone who finds your weight-loss success threatening, you're asking for trouble. You won't be "good old fat so-and-so," someone of no consequence. You have become a powerful person, a winner with positive attitudes whom others may even secretly envy and unknowingly try to sabotage.

Self-acceptance is the state of being a self-reliant person, not dependent on others. Think of how wonderful that will be for you and others too.

Today, stop thinking that self-acceptance involves acceptance by others.

*Today's Action Plan: I will accept myself as a thin, healthy person. I will not let anyone change me back.*

## March 18                                          Have Fun

*Against the assault of laughter, nothing can stand.*
*—Mark Twain*

Winners know how to have fun. True, they are achievers first, but rest and recreation are essential to the positive, productive rhythms of their lives.

Program fun and relaxation into your day along with work, healthy eating, and exercise. You must release pent-up frustration and pressure so that tension doesn't lead to overeating. The accumulation of little irritations can grow into a big problem without a nonfood escape valve.

Take time now to schedule some fun. Fun may be reading, working on a hobby, or being with friends. Make your fun pure pleasure by not mixing it with business. Soon you'll find your stress (and more pounds) melting away.

Relaxation and fun are an essential part of the achiever's life. Today, put your feet up (or get them to a dance floor). Enjoy!

*Today's Action Plan: Today I will do something fun for my well-being. After relaxing, I will be renewed.*

## March 19        Become Your Own Nutritionist

*Jack Sprat could eat no fat, his wife could eat no lean;
And so between the two of them they licked the platter clean.*

—*Mother Goose*

The Sprats knew what they couldn't eat, and you have also learned what to avoid to reach and maintain your healthy weight. Now it's time for you to visit a nutritionist or do research to learn more about how certain nutritional elements work in your body and why.

Once you know how food works in conjunction with organs and glands, you'll learn to listen to what your body is telling you. If you're a sweet-craver, you'll learn to substitute fruit or crunchy vegetables high in natural sugars for nutrient-poor refined sugars. They'll keep your blood sugar levels up so you don't feel that "crash" between meals.

Today, keep an ear tuned to what your body tells you. Learn how food works for you and what to do when it doesn't.

*Today's Action Plan: I will eat energy foods that help me control weight. I accept responsibility for what I eat.*

**March 20**                            **Starving vs. Exercise**

*Diet, Exercise, Attitude.*
*Don't pick one—pick them all.*
           *—Editors of* Executive Fitness Newsletter

Exercise is an essential tool for weight control. In the past, you may have thought you could just cut back on calories and skip all the sweating. But calorie-cutting is no alternative to physical activity.

You may have lost weight fast on low-calorie diets without exercise. But the first thing that happens with calorie restriction alone is that your body uses its glycogen (stored sugar). When you reduce calories, you use your stored energy to run your body. When one pound of glycogen goes, as much as four pounds of water exit with it—not fat, only water. This shows up as your instant weight loss. Next goes protein from muscle tissue, which you want to keep if you intend to look better. And you feel fatigued and become less active, which further slows down fat loss.

Today, recognize the potential harm in the extra-low calorie, no-exercise approach to weight loss.

*Today's Action Plan: I will eat and exercise for health. I will keep an open mind to the idea of exercise.*

*Dieting removes fat only under the most severe prison camp circumstances. A well-exercised body seems to respond more quickly and with less muscle loss.*
                                              *—Covert Bailey*

It takes several weeks for your body to shed fat on a restricted-calorie diet with no exercise. More than twice the calories are stored in a pound of fat than are stored in either a pound of protein or sugar; losing the fat is a slow process by diet alone.

Fat cells reduce their activity in response to famine. If you keep eating less after all the glycogen and muscle protein are gone, your fat cells will protect themselves by burning off much more slowly. Your basal metabolism (the rate calories burn in your body) may slow to almost half its former rate. At this point, if you go off your diet and begin to overeat, you'll gain weight faster than you lost it.

The good news is that you can beat the old lose-gain cycle with exercise. It will speed up your metabolism and your fat will begin to vanish.

Today, learn how your body handles calories. Exercise and diet are perfect partners.

*Today's Action Plan: I will continue to exercise so I can lose weight more successfully. I will embrace the idea of making exercise a habit.*

*Over many thousands of years, since before the dawn of civilization, our bodies have been geared to and sustained by habitual and extensive physical activity.*
                                              *—Dr. Kenneth H. Cooper*

Nature built into your body a wonderful protective device: calorie intake and expenditure automatically adjust to maintain a natural body weight, but only if you are active.

If you exercise reasonably vigorously, your body will continue to burn calories for fifteen hours at a higher rate than it would have without exercise. It's like tuning your car's engine to idle faster—you burn more fuel.

If your metabolism is on the slow side (and it is, if you're an overweight person who's been on and off many diets), regular exercise can boost your metabolism from 20 to 30 percent. That translates into a much lower weight for you.

Today, realize what exercise can do for your body—it gives you a calorie-burning bonus.

*Today's Action Plan: I will raise my metabolism today. I will be body aware.*

**March 23**                    **Exercise to Burn Calories**

*Losing weight was never my problem—I've lost a zillion pounds. But the only way I ever kept it off was putting my body into action.*

*—Georgia Alban*

Now that you're not resisting the idea of exercise quite so much, let's see how you can use it to enhance a high-energy life. First, you'll lose weight faster and be healthier if you exercise. Second, you can control and maintain weight with regular physical exercise.

It is best to split your exercise into two periods, one at the beginning and the other at the end of the day. You don't have to run a marathon or climb the Matterhorn—just twenty minutes of brisk walking will do it. Try alternating three aerobic activities, like bicycling, walking, and jogging (or any other combination) so you won't get bored repeating the same activity each day.

If you should slip off your diet plan, don't berate yourself. Exercise will get rid of those excess calories, producing body heat which literally burns up calories.

Today, accept physical activity as a faster and healthier way to the thin life.

*Today's Action Plan: I will make exercise as much a part of my daily routine as combing my hair. I will take charge of my body.*

**March 24**                                          **Twenty-Five-Hour Day**

*The greatest freedom you have is the freedom to discipline yourself.*
                                        *—Bernard M. Baruch*

A winner's life has a discipline—a winner takes everyday things in stride and builds the daily details into a routine. Establishing a routine for the details of your days means you won't have to make endless decisions about unimportant things. Having disciplined routine squeezes an extra hour out of every day.

Winners get up about the same time every day, eat at the same times, and do all they have to do in about the same number of hours so that they can get proper rest. They have scheduled time for exercise, for healthy eating, and for themselves. They leave time to think and plan for the future. They have time for relaxation and fun, family, and friends.

That might sound boring, but remember what you were like when you were overeating: sick, desperate, tired. You longed for some structure in your life.

Today, decide that the structure of a high-energy, achieving life is what you want. You need never go back to overeating again.

*Today's Action Plan: I will enjoy the freedom of discipline. I will seek it in everyday life.*

## March 25                              You Can Do It

*It is in men as in soils, where sometimes there is a vein of gold, which the owner knows not of.*
— *Jonathan Swift*

Do you believe you can do everything you have to do and 99 percent of what you want to do? For too long you listened to a negative voice in your head that said: "I can't do that. I have no training, or talent, or money." Or even worse, you said, "I'm just not smart enough."

Don't tell yourself that you've tried every diet, every exercise, every doctor, and there's no way out of overeating. This plants a powerful, destructive thought in your head.

Every day, tell yourself that you're ready to adopt new ideas. Break down your old negativity and replace it with a positive, dynamic new self-image. Soon you'll begin to think of yourself as open-minded and quick to master new information. Your mind will begin to filter what you see and hear through the picture of life you need and want.

Today, declare that you are attracted to new ideas, so that new ideas will be attracted to you.

*Today's Action Plan: I will build a new helpful self-image. I will open my mind to the world.*

## March 26                              Now Is the Time

*To everything there is a season, and a time to every purpose under the heaven.*
— *Ecclesiastes 3:1*

This is your season, your day to start becoming the person you want to be. This very second is the time to shift from dependency, to stop relying on food for comfort, and to stop expecting others to tell you who you are. It's time to be an independent, self-reliant adult.

Tell yourself that you have a solution to the problem of overeating that is well within your ability to achieve. Controlling overeating takes constant supervision, but now you have the managerial ability to handle this challenge.

When you overate, your day was likely to be in shambles, your problems overwhelming, and your self-esteem zero. But this is your season. You have let go of overeating as a solution to living problems.

Today, your time has come to accomplish goals. You have enormous reserves of untapped power, and you're going to start using them.

*Today's Action Plan: I will make today the season of my beginning. I will let go of overeating and march ahead to a winner's future.*

## March 27                                                      Luck

*The harder I work, the luckier I get.*

*—Anonymous*

Too many people sit back and wait for luck to knock at their door. Luck really is a change that you have to recognize and be ready for; it's all around you, but you haven't trained yourself to see it.

The more you work at self-understanding, the more you take action on what you learn, and the more ready you will be for luck when it comes your way. For instance, say you find an exciting idea about nutrition. By learning the way your body works, this new idea will mean something special to you. How "lucky" you'll be!

Work hard at the changes you are making in your life. Learn and study and think. You'll get lucky.

Today, see that luck isn't something you fall into, but something you prepare yourself to recognize.

*Today's Action Plan: I will prepare myself to take advantage of every opportunity. I will work hard to make luck a frequent visitor.*

**March 28**                    **Do You Have Binge Foods?**

*I can't drink a little, therefore I never touch it. Abstinence is as easy to me as temperance would be difficult.*

—*Samuel Johnson*

Many of us have foods that we can't control. The first bite leads to countless others, and we are helpless to stop. If you have a binge food, you may have to give it up entirely.

*Giving up binge foods is easier than struggling constantly to control them.* There's no winning with binge foods. One bite is too much and the whole thing isn't enough. Whatever the cause, it's too powerful to control while you're feeding your habit.

Don't try to eat just one. It takes all your energy to stop, and sometimes you can't do it.

Today, discover that it is much easier to get rid of binge foods than to struggle with them in your eating plan.

*Today's Action Plan: I will get rid of my binge foods. I will not allow any food to keep me from greatness.*

*One can never consent to creep when one feels the impulse to soar.*

*—Helen Keller*

You were born to fly, to soar high above the ordinary and average. You have been tied to the ground by your compulsion to overeat too long. If you're creeping instead of flying, the frustration of not doing what you know you can is wrecking your life.

Make a commitment to a thinner body and to the wonderful goals that being overweight has stopped you from achieving. Commitment makes you feel better instantly. Food never did that for you; overeating always made you feel worse.

You don't get something for nothing. It's hard work to develop self-understanding, stay on an eating plan, and exercise regularly. But it's a small price to pay for health, self-confidence, and being in charge of your own life.

Take charge of your own wellness today. There's a price to pay, but the price is nothing compared to the pain of overeating.

*Today's Action Plan: I will put my desire for a healthy, thin body into action. I will soar instead of creep.*

*Adversity has the effect of eliciting talents which, in prosperous circumstances, would have lain dormant.*

*—Horace*

Do you know how lucky you are? You can do something about your overeating right now, today. You're also lucky because the pain of being overweight in a thin-worshipping society has made you stronger than steel.

If you didn't have some steel in you, you wouldn't be the curious and searching person that you are. Many people resist change and act out their negative, destructive habits their whole lives, but you are open to new ideas because you want a life that works.

You may have faults, but a lack of courage isn't one of them. No matter how many times you tried to stop overeating and failed in the past, you have the courage to try again.

Every day you uncover talents you never dreamed you had because you keep on trying. Remember that the next time you are self-critical.

Today, recognize that adversity hasn't destroyed you, but has given you strength and persistence.

*Today's Action Plan: I will not begrudge the pain I've suffered because it uncovered talents I didn't know I had.*

## March 31                    Under the Circumstances

*I am the very slave of circumstance and impulse—borne away with every breath.*

*—Lord Byron*

Without goals that are specifically stated and worked for, overeaters float along without anchors. Any event, good or bad, can be an excuse to overeat. We eat to celebrate; we eat to grieve. Overeating becomes our only response to what happens to us.

Set goals in all areas of your life and make them harmonize with your goal to lose your excess weight and maintain it. Make your goals specific. Tell yourself the number of pounds you want to lose, decide what specific job you want, list the actual improvement you want in your life. Write your goals so that you can see them.

When you stay on your healthy eating plan, you are no slave of circumstances; they don't control you. Today, feel your emotions instead of feeding them, and you will have placed yourself solidly in charge of your life.

*Today's Action Plan: I will take charge of the circumstances of my life. Whatever they are, I will make them better by abstaining from overeating.*

**April 1**                                    **The Worst Vulgarity**

*Habitual vulgarity in an individual is extraordinarily unhealthy, because it mocks the things of the spirit, and slowly squeezes out all serious thought, all fruitful discourse and all genuine sentiment.*

*—Bryan F. Griffin*

Would you make a public joke about someone's height, nose, ears? Of course not. It would be unkind, even vulgar.

That holds especially true for overweight people who abuse *themselves* publicly. *Vulgarity* can apply to people who make themselves the butt of their own fat jokes. "I'm shade in the summer and heat in the winter," announced one woman in front of her friends. "Better guard your good chair," guffawed an overweight man at a party. "I'm gonna kill it!"

The attempt to show people we don't care about our weight by degrading ourselves is the worst vulgarity that can come out of our mouths. It tells others that we see ourselves as clowns and don't take ourselves seriously.

Don't try to make yourself popular at the expense of your dignity. Today, respect yourself. If you don't, no one else will.

*Today's Action Plan: I will not be a jolly fat victim. I will respect myself, especially in front of other people.*

*Life is the thing that really happens to us while we are making other plans.*

—*Anonymous*

There are two ways you can live. The first begins with overeating and trying to manipulate people to gain their approval; it ends in weight gain and loneliness. The second way begins with abstinence from overeating, with a desire for an independent, high-energy life. It ends in fulfillment. The choice, as always, is yours.

Look inside yourself, decide what you want, and begin to work for it. Put your wants into an action plan. You life will agree with your plan, and you'll move in the direction you want to go.

Today, don't let life pass you by. Compare the two ways you can live your life, and choose the one that leads to your happiness.

*Today's Action Plan: I will not allow life just to happen to me. I will make a plan and put it into action.*

*You don't get a second chance to make a first impression.*

—*Vidal Sassoon*

All your life you've been chided—by your mother, by a teacher, by friends—to "put on a happy face." Take that advice today, not so much because your smile might please others, but because it is important to you.

Some overeaters think their faces are only for others to see, but your face also communicates messages to *you.* How do you communicate with your face?

Do you put on a big smile for others and a big frown

for yourself? Are you a man who combs his hair and shaves—for others? Are you a woman who plucks her eyebrows and puts on eye shadow—for others? Then, do you give yourself a scowl?

Choose to send a positive message when you give yourself the first impression of the morning. Start off the day really liking yourself.

Today, put on your best, friendliest, least critical face—for yourself.

> *Today's Action Plan: I will give myself positive messages in my mirror. I will make a good first impression—on me!*

## April 4                                      After Exercise

> *It's your muscles that burn the vast majority of your calories, and even the best diets combined with the most potent vitamins will never tune up your muscles the way good exercise will.*
>
> —*Covert Bailey*

Most exercise-to-expend-calories charts give only part of the story. If you go by the charts, exercise hardly seems worth the trouble. Jog twenty minutes and use only 180 calories—about a glass of milk. Forget it!

But calorie loss isn't the only benefit of exercise. Exercise changes your body's metabolic rate and increases calorie burn long after you stop exercising. Physically fit people who exercise daily burn more calories than sedentary people—even when they're asleep.

Exercise for overweight people is probably more frustrating than dieting ever was, because results are slow. The stored fat won't melt overnight, but it will gradually be replaced by muscle and taut skin.

Today, see the importance of physical exercise in your

total winning program—your body will burn rather than store fat.

*Today's Action Plan: I will exercise my body for physical and emotional satisfaction. I will get the most out of my body today.*

### April 5 Dreams

*If you want your dreams to come true, don't sleep.*
—*Yiddish proverb*

Do you dream of waking up thin one morning? Go ahead and dream, but don't wait passively for your dreams to come true. *Make* them come true.

Believe your dreams. What you can believe, you can achieve.

A thin, healthy body and a winning life are your goals. You can dream of such a happy future, but first cast aside all past failures. You will be free, as if by magic, when you let go of old regrets, recriminations, and excuses.

Tell someone about your dream. The more you hear yourself say it, the more you will believe. It was never dreaming you feared—you were only afraid of failing. That fear grew until it stifled all belief, until the only dreams your mind could conceive were puny and stunted.

Today, don't stifle your great dreams. By believing in your dreams, wonderful things will happen.

*Today's Action Plan: I will unlock my dream power. I will dream dreams of a high-energy life and make them come true.*

*If the only tool you have is a hammer, you tend to see
every problem as a nail.*

—*Abraham Maslow*

When you overate, you were angry with yourself; you
were, as the AA saying goes, "sick and tired of feeling
sick and tired." Every problem was a nail, and your only
response was to hammer on it.

The high-energy life will require a wide array of tools.
Problems will test you, but don't let them arrest you.
Pull your action plan from your repair kit and start to
work. With a positive, constructive attitude, you will
find solutions for obstacles. With anger as your only
tool, you will fail to find solutions. Without solutions,
you may give up—the biggest mistake of all.

If your problem doesn't respond to attitude, reason,
or your action plan, then *you* know you are probably
your problem.

Today, realize that if you have an insoluble problem,
the problem is usually you. Stop hammering on your
problems and learn to work through them.

*Today's Action Plan: Instead of anger, I will use the
power of my mind. I will expand my kit of action
tools.*

*Friend: One who knows all about you and loves you
just the same.*

—*Elbert Hubbard*

Some overeaters pull away from other people fearing
rejection. Theirs is a special loneliness because they
have bought society's fat stereotype and think of them-

selves as passive people to whom things are done, rather than people who do things.

Don't accept the destructive fat stereotype. It's a false image and inconsistent with the winner emerging from within you. But do accept people who want to be your friends, people who can see you as you really are. Don't let your fear of rejection drive others away before you discover their genuine feelings.

If you feel lonely, be a friend. Read the third principle in your action plan: "Radiate warmth." Show others that you care.

Today, reject the idea that overweight people aren't worth knowing. To earn friendship, you have learned you must be a friend.

*Today's Action Plan: I will get rid of my stereotypical fat image. When I'm lonely, I will be a friend to myself and to others.*

**April 8**                                        **A Way Out**

*It is not necessary to hope in order to undertake, nor to succeed in order to persevere.*
                                        —*Blaise Pascal*

You've chosen this book because you know you need help to find a way out of your overeating problem. Your choice reveals that your helplessness and hopelessness have been burned away by your flame of hope.

Your false starts are past—you've discovered a course of action. Don't criticize yourself because it took you so long to reach this day. A winner tries many methods before self-motivation and action lead to victory.

When you take action instead of waiting for others to, you take control of your direction. You move forward, like a winner. Temporary adjustments may be needed along the way, but you will continue your weight control program. Your determination to persevere feels good.

Today, see that a flame of hope still burns within you.

*Today's Action Plan: I will cherish the bright flame of hope. I will be a victor, not a victim.*

## April 9                                    You're No Invalid

*The stock approach to the fat person is to start him on a diet as the first order of business and to worry about the rest later, and of course, "later" never really comes.*
*—Dr. William Bennett*

Have you repeatedly started an exercise program, but couldn't stick to it? You may have subconsciously thought of yourself as an invalid, someone who is incapable of physical exercise.

Western medicine has traditionally seen dieting as the "cure" to being overweight. Since most diet-only programs are unsuccessful, other kinds of health care such as exercise and attitude change never seem to get started. Overweight patients are then seen as chronic failures and, as such, invalids.

Unfortunate as the stereotype may be, we perceive invalids as those who restrict their activities and remove themselves from circulation. Even the word *invalid* means "without worth."

Are you seeing yourself as an invalid? Today, begin perceiving yourself as a physical person instead. Understanding is the basis for action.

*Today's Action Plan: I will prove that I am not an invalid. I will discover the active person within me.*

*Actions speak louder than words.*

*—Old saying*

Action is character. You may argue that character is a combination of personality traits, good and bad. But people are what they do—not what they say. A man with a dry sense of humor makes wry comments. A woman with a reputation for honesty tells the truth. Only through acts do we know ourselves and others.

Character isn't set in concrete, no matter how old your habits are. Your negative habits—overeating, eating unhealthy foods, and avoiding physical activity—can be replaced with positive new actions and habits.

What you do is what you are. Yesterday's habits are replaced by today's action. Today you can and will do things that will change your character.

Today, take a step toward changing your character by doing what you want to become. Action leads directly to the thinner, high-energy life you want.

*Today's Action Plan: I will do what it takes to become who I want to be. I will replace old behavior with something new.*

*I blamed everything but me for being fat. It was my way of denying that I had a need I couldn't fill.*

*—Jerri Hannah*

Anyone who sincerely wants to get out of the fat trap can escape by increasing self-understanding—by realizing that change is possible and developing a plan for change. But before you can have self-understanding, you have to get rid of all the lies you believe—like your inability to lose weight.

We overeaters lie to ourselves. As self-deceivers, we deny the reality of what we're doing to our lives. But when the pain breaks through, reality is there staring us in the face.

Embrace reality. Self-deception feeds on fresh lies every day; self-understanding is nurtured by what is real and true. When you stop lying to yourself about who you are and what you want, self-deception will vanish from the scene.

Today, face your life as it is, without pretense. Self-understanding and self-deception can't coexist if you're going to be honest with yourself.

*Today's Action Plan: I will tell myself the truth. I'll embrace reality so my actions will take me where I want to go.*

## April 12        Try Again, Now that You've Changed

*We are new every day.*
          —*Irene Claremont de Castillego*

When we change, we don't always realize it. We may continue to act in old, habitual ways. Shyness, particularly if carried over from childhood, is one of the traits we often keep.

A capable government engineer was required to attend meetings, during which he always remained silent. When the meetings ended, he hurried away. When asked why he never contributed, he said, "I've been shy in groups since I was a boy." Hearing this, a new man in the department laughed and said, "You, shy? Why, you're the most competent man here."

During the next meeting, the engineer voluntarily explained a complicated plan without a stumble. The only difference was his action. He'd stopped being shy long ago, he just hadn't discovered it. His shyness was a habit of thinking, not a fact.

Do you have some habitual behavior that makes you say: "Oh, no. I can't"? Is it no longer relevant? Today, discard fixed thinking that no longer applies to you.

*Today's Action Plan: I will do what I've convinced myself I couldn't do. I will take the first opportunity to try my wings.*

### April 13                                    It's No Sin

*Eating has become the last bona fide sin.*
                                        —*Ellen Goodman*

Overweight isn't immoral and thinness isn't moral. Good and bad have nothing to do with overeating. When you finally understand this, you'll be able to put recrimination behind you.

As an overweight person, you must withstand our culture's thin-is-in attitudes of blame, loathing, and mockery. As the tenth principle in your action plan says, "Reject rejection firmly and totally," from others and from yourself.

Every day you are building a dynamic image of yourself, so don't predict your own failure, don't laugh at your goals, don't allow anyone to deter you from your new life. *You* are in charge.

Today, understand that being overweight is not a moral problem, but one of attitude, right-eating, and exercise.

*Today's Action Plan: I will not think of myself as a sinner, but as someone with a health problem that I'm doing something about.*

*You know not how to live in clover.*

                     *—Menander*

As bad as your life was when you ate compulsively—when food, not you, was in charge—at least the routine was familiar: binge, regret, diet, slip, binge. That destructive cycle was so much a part of your daily existence that you couldn't imagine any other. You even feared diet success because it was unknown.

Your old life was built around the false joy of overeating. Now that you've found a dynamic new lifestyle, you've lost the imagined pleasure of overeating, as well as pounds and pain. Food is no longer at the center of your life. Success is your new center.

Think of the positive things you can do to fill the vacuum left by the absence of your food obsession. Winners who *get rid* of pounds and pain can fill up with success.

Today, acknowledge that fear of diet success is simply a fear of the unknown. The pain of overeating is too high a price to pay for maintaining familiar old patterns.

*Today's Action Plan: I will know that losing my food obsession is not deprivation, but privilege. I will fill any emptiness with my new winner's attitude.*

*People can be divided into three groups: those who make things happen, those who watch things happen, and those who wonder what happened.*

                     *—Yiddish proverb*

Winners dare to make their dreams become reality; they have the audacity to go into action and get what they want. When are you going to make your desires become real? Immediately.

A slender body is a natural desire; it is perfectly natural to want it. Take the time to nurture this desire. Visualize it. Commit yourself to achieving the body you want. An element of risk exists, but without risk there can be no success. Convince yourself that you can succeed.

In which of the three groups do you want to belong? Do you want to watch the parade go by? Do you want to be out of control and wonder what happened? Or do you want to make things happen?

Today, choose the group you belong in and dare to go for it.

*Today's Action Plan: I will make things happen. I will begin now.*

## April 16                                    Getting Even

*Success is the best revenge.*

—*French proverb*

If you were an overweight child, you may be haunted by childhood memories of schoolyard bullies. As an overweight adolescent, you remember being excluded from the fun of teen years. Now, as an overweight adult, you may face discrimination on the job and ridicule by society. You may have a right to be angry, but instead, choose success. That's the best way to put ugly memories to rest.

You're not a weight, you're an important human being. You have made health a goal because you want a high-energy, in-control life. You want to feel great, look wonderful in your clothes, and deal with your weight problem successfully so that you can experience your life fully.

Today, erase ugly memories by filling the rest of your life with achievement.

*Today's Action Plan: I will lose weight because I want to get more out of life. After all the laughter and cruelties, I will achieve a unique place in this world.*

## April 17                                              Less Is More

*People have to be informed and more aware of nutrients in foods, so that they can make intelligent individual choices.*

—*Dr. Kathleen Zolber*

As you choose an eating plan for weight loss and better health, it's a good idea to learn more about your own nutritional needs. Very likely, you'll learn to cut back on sugar, fat, and salt in your eating program.

Abusing these three substances can cause a host of physical problems, as well as slow down weight loss and maintenance. For a healthier lifestyle, follow these basic rules:

- Limit fat by reducing high-fat dairy foods, saturated oils, and red meat.
- Limit salt by adding only small amounts for cooking and none at the table. Reduce or eliminate salty snack foods.
- Limit refined sugar by reducing or eliminating sweets.

You already know which foods need to be reduced or eliminated from your diet. Now put your knowledge into action.

Today, learn more about nutrition so you can make wise food decisions. As you reduce the negative effects of food each day, you increase food's positive uses for your good health.

*Today's Action Plan: I will reduce or eliminate salt, fat, and sugar. I will say yes to good nutrition.*

**April 18**                                    **Taking Inventory**

*When growth ceases, decay and decline begin.*
                                    *—Henry Clay Lindgren*

Do you have a blaming, prejudicial attitude toward your weight? That's a self-hateful way to live. If you want to help yourself make your life work better, concentrate on self-help.

Take inventory of your positive attributes. You have many marvelous qualities buried under your negative self-image. Take them out, look at them, and say, "I'm a good person. I don't have any reason to be ashamed."

The next time you bad-mouth yourself, stop and point to one of your positive qualities instead. You weren't embarrassed to say unkind things about yourself in the past, so don't be embarrassed to say nice things to yourself now.

Today, see how you have treated yourself worse than you would allow anyone else to treat you. Decide not to harass yourself any longer.

*Today's Action Plan: From now on, I will replace my self-criticism with my positive program of self-understanding, diet, and exercise.*

**April 19**                                    **A Powerful Motivator**

*Recognition: an acknowledgment.*
                                    *—Webster's Unabridged Dictionary*

A motivator is something people respond to on a gut level. Powerful motivators drive us to our goals, and one of the most powerful of all motivators is recognition.

Compulsive personalities—the kind many overeaters have—seem to demand more approval from the world than the world is willing to give. We manipulate pleasing people to make them say that we're important to them. And we may be successful praise-wheedlers for a time, but negative inner voices keep telling us how unworthy we are.

You're absolutely right to want recognition, but no one can hand it to you. On the other hand, action equals achievement, which equals recognition. It also creates a wonderful feeling of security and satisfaction.

Today, you've learned the right way to earn the acknowledgment you've always wanted.

*Today's Action Plan: I will seek recognition through achievement. I will aim for goals that demand achievement.*

## April 20                    Be Prepared to Walk Alone

*Alone, alone, all, all alone;*
*Alone on a wide, wide sea!*
                    *—Samuel Taylor Coleridge*

If you make a commitment to high performance and real achievement, you'll have to accept one of the consequences of that commitment—being alone.

Perhaps you won't be as available to others as in the past. You may even have to say no when you are asked to do something that might jeopardize your recovery.

Ultimately you have to stand alone. You have friends, family, fellow weight-losers, co-workers, and others who wish you well, but when you stand toe-to-toe, slugging it out with temptation, you fight alone. When no one can help you but yourself, you have to be ready.

Now that you are committed to healthy goals, you'll

have energy for others that you didn't have before, but don't forget to take care of yourself. Say no, when you must, to protect your commitment.

Today, put personal commitment to achievement before pleasing others. Do this so you can be of real use to yourself and ultimately to others.

*Today's Action Plan: I will stand alone to protect my commitment when I must. I will resolve not to jeopardize my recovery from overeating.*

## April 21                                    Your Own Way

*They are able because they think they are able.*
                                                —*Virgil*

One way to rid yourself of a hurtful compulsion is to develop a helpful one. Freedom from overeating can be a helpful compulsion. Getting rid of the compulsion to overeat is not easy, but overeating causes you pain, and you want to rid yourself of the pain to gain self-control. Self-control is another name for freedom from food.

The freedom of self-discipline is a real freedom. It brings security, stability, self-understanding, and achievement. You can develop a positive craving for the freedom of self-discipline, and when you have it, there is no room in your life for other compulsions.

Today, see that out-of-control eating is not freedom, but the worst kind of slavery. The freedom of self-discipline is the freedom you crave.

*Today's Action Plan: I will be free of my food compulsion. I will fight through to a winner's self-control.*

*We may our ends by our beginnings know.*
                     —*Sir John Denham*

The longest journey, as the Chinese proverb says, begins with the first step, so make that step a good one. Don't say, "I'll try." Say, "I'll do it." Action is commitment.

Since you are a new person every day, you must renew your commitment every day. Each day, as you read this book, commit yourself to living without excess food. If you had a slip yesterday, give yourself another chance today—give yourself a thousand chances. The only failure is in punishing yourself for a stumble, self-destructively taking away a new chance for a positive life.

Beginnings and endings are related; if you want a happy ending, make a happy beginning. Go joyously to work on yourself.

Today, give yourself a good beginning, which is the first step to a happy ending. One good step at a time, one good day at a time, can change your life.

*Today's Action Plan: I will recommit myself to a winner's life. I will make a good beginning.*

*The whole is greater than the sum of its parts.*
                   —*General systems theory*

If you've never studied physics, you've missed an idea that could be useful to you—the general systems theory. Overeaters are often impatient people; we want what we want, and we want it *right now*. We've got every right to yearn for the good life, but achievement is the result of putting all the right parts together so the whole emerges.

All the little parts of the winning puzzle that you read about so far are necessary to the whole. No principle in your action plan is the answer by itself, but all of them together make a whole winning life possible. Read them over at least once a day, especially if you're feeling frustrated and vulnerable. Review them so you can check to see that you're still on course.

Today, see the relationship of all the small parts of your plan to the whole. Each one is important to complete the picture of your success.

*Today's Action Plan: I will remember that all the parts of my winning plan have to be in place before the whole picture emerges. I will read the principles of my action plan.*

**April 24**  **Who's Responsible for Your Weight?**

*It is in the ability to deceive oneself that the greatest talent is shown.*

—*Anatole France*

There are a hundred theories about how people become overweight. It doesn't matter which one eventually proves to be correct. Right now, today, you are responsible for your weight. You, and only you, can deal with it—not your doctor, your family, your friends, or members of your support group.

Why should you be happy about this? If others are responsible for your weight, then someone or something is in control of your life. If you are responsible, then you are in control. You control your life—no one and nothing but you.

What does having control mean? It means that what

you think and what you do control the way you feel. Winners base their entire lives on this concept. You can too.

Today, own yourself. You are ready to take the mystery out of achievement and put in your own control.

*Today's Action Plan: I will own my weight. I will accept help, but when it comes to doing, it's all up to me.*

## April 25                                    The Right Moves

*We are creatures of habit. So let the force of habit help you maintain your exercise program.*
        —*Dr. Kenneth H. Cooper*

Are you making the right moves? Weight maintenance is based on the laws of thermodynamics—energy in equals energy out. So why not put more emphasis on the energy-out side of the equation?

There's another aspect of exercise you may not have considered. Exercise changes your self-image from an immobile, sedentary person to an active, moving person. Visualize yourself running, jogging, swimming, bicycling. You're exhilarated and you look great!

The average person, regardless of weight, doesn't stick to exercise. But you're not average. And you know vigorous exercise helps you lose weight even if you don't lower your food intake. Find an exercise program that works for you and stick to it.

Today, look at the energy equation and decide to be on the side of the winners.

*Today's Action Plan: I will make the right moves. I will be one of the winners in life.*

*Anger is a short madness.*

*—Horace*

Of all the emotional energy available to overeaters, anger is often the most ill-spent. In this world full of frustrations, anger is a normal reaction. How can we handle that legitimate anger in constructive ways?

First, be prepared for less-than-perfect treatment from others. It's not always a fair world, and when you realize this, you won't be outraged when someone is inconsiderate.

Second, don't turn your anger on yourself. When something goes wrong, it isn't always your fault. Turning your anger inward is a way to avoid confronting others, but the results are disastrous.

If your anger is appropriate, face the source of your anger. Tell your oppressor, "I don't like that." The negative things that happen to you are not your fault because you are overweight. You have a right to be angry, but also a responsibility to express it constructively.

Today, confront anger instead of letting it simmer. Your weight has nothing to do with your rights to human feelings of frustration.

*Today's Action Plan: I will not expect the world to treat me with kid gloves. I will not turn anger against myself.*

*I may be unhappy with myself, but at least I'm never bored while I'm eating.*

*—Overheard at a diet group*

You have an enemy that can destroy the best action plan for right-eating: boredom. It is a villain lurking on every overeater's path to achievement, but you can turn this trap into a triumph.

Overeaters often eat to excess to fill time. Unfilled time allows too much opportunity for unpleasant emotions to surface. Thoughts of unmet responsibilities and a hundred guilts and fears can rise up to haunt you. But eating is no way to resolve negative feelings about yourself.

It's hard to be bored if you are following the action-filled life demanded by the achiever's schedule. You're just too busy. The achieving life is crammed to the brim with positive mental and physical activity. Winners are seldom bored.

Today, see that boredom is really empty time filled with negative feelings and behavior. Action, on the other hand, is never boring.

*Today's Action Plan: I will be too busy to be bored. Boredom is an excuse to overeat, and I will not use this excuse again.*

## April 28 — Never Too Tired

*At the end of the day, I was too tired to prepare the proper foods.*
*— Overheard at a diet group*

Winners plan ahead. You are serious about losing weight, so you give your eating and exercise plan top priority. Make the foods you need to eat easily available so you won't grab high-calorie snacks to get over the fatigue slump.

Ignoring your need for the food on your plan does not de-emphasize food. Instead, it sabotages your program. When you're tired, the temptation to reach for the nearest food is far stronger than when you're rested.

Schedule some relaxation time into every day. This prevents you from getting so tired that you resort to the old food pacifier. If you are getting too tired to maintain smart eating habits, change your schedule.

Most of us convince ourselves that we save time by grabbing the first food at hand. Too often this means slipping into a binge. But the binge-guilt pattern never saves time.

Today, plan ahead and keep the foods you need close at hand. You're acting more like a winner every day.

*Today's Action Plan: I will not allow myself to get too tired. I will not use fatigue as an excuse to overeat.*

## April 29          Never Too Hungry

*I skipped breakfast, and by lunch I was ready to eat everything in the house.*
*—Diet club member*

Many dieters think if they're not hungry, the diet isn't working. This is as silly as believing a medicine won't cure if it isn't bitter. If you have a nutritionally balanced eating plan, you should be hungry at mealtimes, but not too hungry.

Don't skip meals. Nothing—absolutely nothing—is more important to your high-energy life than nourishing, tasty meals.

Listen to your body. Don't try to set some arbitrary time for meals that doesn't correspond to your body's needs. If your family has to eat earlier or later, let them, at least until you can gradually wean your body from its preferred time.

For an overeater, getting too hungry is dangerous. Take whatever steps you must to avoid it.

Today, do what you must to achieve your goals. You have a winner's curiosity and determination.

*Today's Action Plan: I will not allow myself to get too hungry. I will plan meals so I won't have an excuse to overeat.*

**April 30**                                   **Where You Are and**
                                               **Where You're Going**

*Milestone: an important event or turning point.*
                                   —Webster's Dictionary

One third of the year has passed. How has it gone for you? Have you let it slip away one day at a time, taking with it forgotten or broken promises that you made to yourself? Or have you fanned your little pilot light of hope into a fire that has warmed your life and lighted your way to achievement?

Each day your dream is alive. It's just as strong today as it was on January 1. Each day you are new. And you are capable.

A life of overeating suffocates. It has consequences that have names: grief, confusion, anger, guilt. A winning, achieving life has fantastic rewards that have names, too: self-esteem, self-understanding, confidence, courage, authority.

The choice is yours. It will be your choice every day of this year, every day of your life. Only you can truly put your plan into action. Have you made that decision?

Today, keep the light of hope glowing. You have the ability, now put it into action.

*Today's Action Plan: I will fan the flame of hope, and say yes to a winner's life.*

**May 1**                                 **A Debt You Don't Owe**

*Worry is interest paid on trouble before it falls due.*
            *—William Ralph Inge*

We overeaters are often overworriers, especially when our eating is out of control. We tend to "terrible-ize" the future because the present is so awful. Our self-destructive negative fantasies destroy our chances for success.

When you worry about imaginary trouble, you believe in false limits. You live in a world closed to achievement. On the other hand, if you always expect to win, you increase the odds in your favor.

You've got work to do today: uncover a layer of self-deception, give up a negative illusion, expose a false fear. Don't stand still while your life marches by. Use your imprisoned energy to get into action.

Today, face worry and discard the limitations you have inflicted on yourself.

*Today's Action Plan: I will not "terrible-ize" the future. I will not limit my life with false fears.*

**May 2**                                     **The Big Sell-Out!**

*One is never too old to yearn.*

            *—Italian proverb*

Have you ever said, "If I were younger, I could lose weight," or, "If I were older, I could control my overeating"? If so, you used age as an excuse for not making a commitment to losing weight.

Age is no barrier to a winning life. You can get the action habit at sixteen or sixty. Being a winner can mean more admiration, self-esteem, and respect, and less fear, failure, and worries. Winning brings happiness and satisfaction to your life, and you're never too old or too young for those benefits.

Failure is fed by excuses; winning is fed by knowing and doing what's important to you. You know what's important to you today.

Don't let age be a ticket to a self-limited life. Get the action habit today, whatever your age.

*Today's Action Plan: I will not allow age to be a barrier to my goals. I am the perfect age to win.*

**May 3**                   **The Advance Guard of Winning**

*The first principle of achievement is mental attitude. Man begins to achieve when he begins to believe.*
                                        —*J. C. Roberts*

You can't wish away extra pounds, but you can believe them away. Strong belief in a goal propels you into action, and your belief communicates confidence to others. They feed this positive energy back to you, further increasing your belief in yourself.

Believe you will succeed. Believe you will lose weight, take charge of your life, and get on the winner's path. Look at the really successful people around you. Chances are they aren't smarter than you, nor do they have any secret door open for them. The difference is their powerful belief that they will succeed.

Begin to believe that nothing can keep you overweight. This one basic belief will power your mind.

Your mind will then begin to attract and develop answers.

Today, believe—it's the most positive power you can use. Like perpetual motion, your belief sends out waves of confidence that come back as others' belief in you.

*Today's Action Plan: I believe I can lose weight. I know I can keep a healthy weight as long as I believe.*

### May 4                                    Yesterday's Ghosts

*Until you learn to name your ghosts and to baptize your hopes, you have not yet been born; you are still the creation of others.*
*—Marie Cardinal*

Name your ghosts. When you learn what your fears are, you can recognize your hopes. Then, free from fear and armed with legitimate hope, you can re-create yourself. You can be reborn in a new likeness, in a new body and mind that you will be proud of.

There is a place that only your unique self can fill. Imagine yourself in that place. Accept today's hopes and recognize the effort you put into today's improvement.

Above all, on this day, respect yourself. You are uniquely wonderful; no one else in this world can be like you. Because you try, each day you win a little more. Name yesterday's fears: call them indecision, bingeing, lack of goals. They are only ghosts.

Today, encourage yourself as only you can. You have named your fears and they are gone.

*Today's Action Plan: I will get rid of the fear ghosts. I will baptize my hope in commitment to goals.*

*We shall not cease from exploration.*

*—T. S. Eliot*

You can find assets in unexpected places that will help you reach your goals. The next time you start criticizing yourself, look at your supposed liabilities with a positive eye.

Let's say you are a fussy housekeeper. That's not necessarily negative. You are also very exact. When you haven't a goal to work toward, you may be fussy for the sake of fussiness. When you have a goal—such as a healthy body—your behavior changes from fussiness to exactness. Your behavior is focused toward your goal.

If you tend to become negatively overinvolved, a goal will transform that liability into the asset of focused energy. If you are angry, a goal will transform that into assertiveness. Possibilities arise when you look at yourself positively.

Today, by adding a goal, turn character problems into assets. Goals can turn a self-defeating course into a path to the winner's circle.

*Today's Action Plan: I will turn my liabilities into assets. I will look at the positive side of my behavior.*

*We act ourselves into ways of believing and believe ourselves into ways of acting.*

*—Joseph Chilton*

Thinking is preparation for action. But action must follow thought or the thought is wasted. "I'll think about this weight goal," you say. But thinking isn't action.

Think, decide, then act. Take specific action. Create opportunities for success whether your goal is ten pounds or one hundred pounds.

There's a risk of failure with commitment, but dare to take that risk. Failing only means you have more to learn; it doesn't mean you're finished. If you've stumbled, you've learned something.

Predict success, keep believing, and you will reach your weight goal. Nothing can stop you.

Today, go beyond thinking and trying to action. Commitment together with action is the only way to achieve your goal.

*Today's Action Plan: I will take action on my weight goal. I will risk anything but the risk of not beginning.*

**May 7**                                    **The Sugar Monster**

*The more sugar you eat in a lifetime, the more abnormal your response to sugar becomes.*
                                                  *—Dr. Robert Atkins*

Are you hooked on refined sugar? Does one bite of a sweet mean that you'll probably eat to the bottom of the container?

Do you use sugar as emotional therapy, running to it as to a lover, friend, or comforter whenever you're under stress? After eating a lot of refined sugar, do you have headaches, drowsiness, bloating, weeping spells, a hungover feeling the next day? What is your body telling you?

If you were just an average sweet-user and could cut out refined sugar for one year, you would rid your body of the caloric equivalent of fifty pounds. If sugar is a real problem for you, getting rid of it completely is the only way to bring your craving under control.

Today, face the fact that refined sugar is a barrier to the kind of achieving life you want.

*Today's Action Plan: I will evaluate honestly what my body is telling me about refined sugar. If I need to, I will cut myself off from sugar.*

## May 8                                   What Do You Want?

*What you should want more than the habit is the benefit of giving it up.*

—*José Silva*

What do you want more than anything? Do you wish to lose weight and maintain your weight goal, to become a winner for the rest of your life?

Your wish will be granted if you follow seven basic, powerful ideas. Don't be fooled by their simplicity; they will take all your strength to achieve.

1. Define what you want.
2. Live intensely with that idea.
3. Become thin in your own mind first.
4. Visualize yourself at your natural weight.
5. Let go of negative emotional baggage.
6. Practice consistent positive affirmation.
7. Put it all into action.

Do you recognize the power in these ideas? If you do what it takes, you will become the person you want to become.

Today, state what you want. These powerful ideas can open the world of achievement to you.

*Today's Action Plan: I will define what I want to be. Then I will win.*

*Self-reverence, self-knowledge, self-control,*
*These three alone lead life to sovereign power.*
                                          *—Alfred, Lord Tennyson*

Pop psychology aside, nobody else can hand you self-esteem: not a parent, not a mate, not a friend. Only *you* can give yourself self-esteem. Like yourself. That's all there is to it.

Now, how do you go about liking yourself? This, too, is not complex. Self-esteem means you are happily involved with yourself—not morbidly or obsessively, as in the past, but happily as you are right now.

Because you have a weight problem, you may need to change your pattern of thinking about yourself. Whisper it, so that someday you may shout it: "I like myself!"

Today, see how liking yourself is inextricably linked with how effective you are. And that determines how well you will lose weight and keep it off.

*Today's Action Plan: I will build up my self-esteem, liking myself more today than I did yesterday. I will know what it is to love myself.*

*Without discipline, one can only stare like a window-shopper at the good things in life, and shrug, and move on.*

                                          *—Amy Gross*

A photographer has a trick for getting people to smile for the camera. "If you love sex," he shouts, "smile!" Invariably a grin spreads across the subject's face. If the photographer had substituted *discipline* for *sex* those portraits might have been more grim. But if *you* stepped into the picture, you'd grin for discipline.

When you stopped overeating and began to achieve the winning life, you realized that daily discipline was necessary to your happiness. A major ingredient of your success was a structured life.

You found there is nothing more comforting and comfortable than a day based on doing what you know you should do, when you know you should do it.

Today, reinforce your own daily discipline and put structure into your day to make it better. The way to achieve what you want is to go after it systematically.

*Today's Action Plan: I will be a disciplined doer, not a window-shopper in life. I will love a structured day.*

## May 11                                         Disguised

*Without my magic cloak of blubber and invisibility, I felt naked, pruned as though some essential covering was missing.*

                                         —Margaret Atwood

One of the awful mysteries of being overweight is losing excess weight—even hundreds of pounds—only to regain it all and then some. This is the infamous yo-yo syndrome, with the yo-yo bouncing back ever higher. Nothing is more painful than the hopelessness and shame of regaining all your lost weight.

Yet, some people who have experienced this did not feel comfortable with their bodies when they were thin. The longer they were overweight, the harder it was to lose the fat self-image.

One way to prevent the yo-yo syndrome is to convince yourself that you deserve to be thin. Now is the time to discard your overweight self-image and develop a solid understanding of your unique worth. And it is possible when you approach your new lifestyle with attention and concentration.

Today, see the necessity of adjusting your inner image, so it will be comfortable with the new thin body you will have.

*Today's Action Plan: I will not hide inside my excess pounds. My inner mirror will reflect my true image.*

## May 12                                    Get a Mentor

*If you want success, copy from someone.*
— *W. Clement Stone*

People in the business world offer mutual support by networking—working with supportive people who can help them make good career decisions. Often there is one special person who can guide them to success: a mentor. Successful diet groups have mentors, or sponsors. They give encouragement, direction, and strength to fellow overeaters.

Successful people are easy to recognize. They don't talk a good job, they do a good job; they don't just think about losing weight, they lose weight. They are people you can honestly admire because they've turned their lives around.

Choose a good mentor (or more than one) and then imitate their success, adapting their methods to your needs.

Today, set out toward success by seeking doers and imitating them.

*Today's Action Plan: I will find a mentor. I will listen to what he or she tells me, and do it.*

*The future belongs to those who live intensely in the present.*

                                                   *—Anonymous*

Twelve Step groups such as Alcoholics Anonymous, which offer hope and recovery to people addicted to alcohol and other drugs, food, gambling, and so on, teach that no one can live any time except now.

Far too many compulsive people try to live in every time but the present. They drag yesterday's mistakes around and worry about repeating them tomorrow. Today is totally lost while they fret about the past and fear the future. Life passes them by, a day at a time.

Today is the only day you can do anything about. By the time you go to bed tonight, be one day closer to achieving a thinner body, self-understanding, and a high-energy, enthusiastic life. Create a chance for yourself by concentrating all your desire into the next few hours.

Today, release yesterday and tomorrow and focus on this day. You can use each day only once.

*Today's Action Plan: I will take life one day at a time. At the end of the day, I will be closer to my goal.*

*Believe you can, or believe you can't; either way you'll be right.*

                                                 *—Henry Ford*

You can respond two ways to a compliment: with self-affirmation or self-criticism. When a friend says, "You were great!" you can say, "Thank you," or "Oh, that's nothing." Which do you want: an inner criticizer or a inner affirmer?

Don't brush aside compliments as if they were of no consequence. Accept the validation of others. Believe you are worthy.

Your criticizer erodes your self-esteem when you tell yourself, "You're so stupid!" Be more self-encouraging. Tell yourself, "I am fun to be around," or, "I really did a great job that time." It's important to give yourself the compliments you richly deserve.

Today, listen to your self-affirmer. Tell yourself, "I'm doing a great job putting my weight-loss plan into action. I'm a winner."

*Today's Action Plan: I will overwhelm my criticizer with self-affirmation. I will compliment myself at least once today.*

## May 15                    The Success of Failure

*We are all failures—at least the best of us are.*
        *—Sir James M. Barrie*

No matter how hard people try, they sometimes fail. Overeaters know this all too well. How many times have you said, "I've failed again"?

Don't view failure as a catastrophe that happens only to you. Failure is part of playing to win. If you get in the game, you might drop the ball.

Never see a failure as losing the whole ballgame. View it as simply gaining information you need to change your methods. Failure is just a new set of instructions to help you reach your goal.

Value the chance a failure gives you to perfect your action plan. It's an opportunity to practice your positive mental techniques and perfect your performance for the next confrontation.

Today, squeeze success out of failure. Learn what you can from failure, so that the next time you'll be wiser and tougher.

*Today's Action Plan: I will find a new way to look at failure. I will focus on the positive future, not the negative past.*

**May 16**                             **Yes, You Can Do More**

*Do more than exist, live.*

—*John H. Rhoades*

Are you doing all you can to get a thin, healthy body? There is no limit to how much you can improve. Successful people have a simple formula for daily achievement: Do what you do well even better, and try to do even more of it every day.

Do more than notice your feelings about overeating; understand them. Do more than read about nutrition; make this knowledge a part of you. Do more than hear; listen for meaning. Do more than think; put your thoughts into action.

You can do all these things. What you want, you can achieve. What you desire, you deserve. Your life will be better if that's what you want.

Today, become an achiever. Don't put limits on success; believe you can do a little more each day to build a whole new life.

*Today's Action Plan: I will do what I do well even better. I will do a little more of it today.*

*Fat people often think of themselves solely in terms of the "neck up." Their bodies are disowned, alienated, foreign, perhaps stubbornly present but not truly a part of the real self.*
—*Marcia Millman*

Does shopping for clothes make you realize how much you hate your body? If so, you are cooperating with your inner critic's campaign to bring you down.

You are important enough to look your best every day, no matter what your present weight. So dress as if today will be the most successful day of your life.

You need to look important to others, so they will mirror that back to you. But even more, you need to look important for yourself. A good appearance helps you to think on a higher level, to risk more, to change more. When you look in the mirror, your image should say: "You are important, intelligent, and achieving."

Today, dress to reflect how important you are.

*Today's Action Plan: I will honor myself by dressing well today.*

*One of these days is none of these days.*
—*Henry George Bohn*

People who constantly mutter, "If only . . . ," have never learned to give themselves a next time. They are stuck in regret, unable to see the opportunities around them.

You've got work to do today. You have a goal to pursue, a plan to put into action, an idea to work on, a problem to solve, a decision to make. You are too busy *doing* to be an "If only" person.

Using the present is the admission ticket to a full life. Get rid of your favorite excuses for postponing living—lack of money, support, talent, tools. You have all you need—the desire to achieve a whole life, to be a thinner winner.

Today, refuse to poison your life with "If only." That is the cry of dreams never launched, goals never pursued, projects never started.

*Today's Action Plan: I will not postpone a minute of my life. I will take action now to get where I want to go.*

**May 19**                    **A Two-Minute Picture of You**

*He who values himself is valued.*

*—Anonymous*

Practice your action plan and you will gain a new best friend: yourself. Our self-esteem often gets so low that it's difficult to do good things for ourselves. But today treat yourself like a new person.

- Act as if you value, not hate, yourself; as if you understand, not despise, yourself.
- Act as if you are poised, not tense; confident, not confused; bold, not timid.
- Act as if you are full of enthusiasm, not bored; achieving, not failing; energized, not tired.
- Act as if you are a positive person, and you will become as you act.

The game of "acting as if" works. You don't even have to believe at first; doing will create belief. Your dreams will come true when you really become your own best friend.

Today, act as if you already have everything you need to create a thinner, healthier body. You do!

*Today's Action Plan: I will value myself. I will act out and believe in this positive picture of myself.*

*The best way to make your dreams come true is to wake up.*

—*George Alban*

If your biggest dream is to reach and maintain your natural weight, your dream can come true. One of the basic principles of action (incorporated in the twelfth principle of your action plan) is "always play to win." When your creative energies are propelled by a winning dream, you can get going and keep going.

First, you must love yourself enough to give yourself your dream. Then you must put that dream into action. If you play life to win, your dreams come true.

Winning begins with hope, but you must supply the action to motivate it. Do you hope you can be free from the nightmare of overeating and will wake up to a happy, winning life? Soon this hope will come true.

Today, be awake to your dreams and use them to fuel action. You want to lose your excess weight and play life to win.

*Today's Action Plan: I will put my dreams into action. I will win my fondest dream.*

*There is no upper limit to what individuals are capable of doing with their minds.*

—*E. F. Wells*

Success is usually defined as the attainment of personal goals—but not just a weight goal. Most overeaters need to make big changes in attitude, outlook, and the way they respond to life. Goals that include an improved outlook on life can help you uncover a powerful person within you, one whom you didn't know existed.

You are making an investment in the present that will change your future. You are building an action program of exercise, attitude, and right-eating for weight loss.

Today, you will travel as far as your inner ability will take you, and that is a great distance. You have no upper limit.

Today, expand your definition of success as far as your commitment—endlessly.

*Today's Action Plan: I will define what success means to me. I will open myself to change.*

## May 22                                          All or Nothing

*Failure is a teacher—a harsh one, but the best.*
*—Thomas J. Watson Jr.*

Do you know any all-or-nothing people? One little mistake can lead them to abandon an entire project. If you are such a person, one little bite can lead to an overeating binge. All-or-nothingism is a defeating mind-set.

If you take a bite of a food you've decided to eliminate from your diet, it's no reason to go all the way; it's a reason to look for the reason. Analyze that failure and make it work for you. Knowing why you made an eating misstep will arm you if the same problem arises again.

Small mistakes don't ruin your life any more than a single bite ruins your fine eating plan. Think of mistakes as a form of quick education and learn from them. You'll reach your life's goals faster.

Today, let go of the all-or-nothing habit. You're a quick learner!

*Today's Action Plan: I will profit from my mistakes. I will learn from every misstep.*

**May 23**                    **Why Do You Binge?**

*First I made a mental list of all the "goodies" I'd been sacrificing on my diet. Then I proceeded to eat my way through the whole list.*
                                        *—Diet group member*

This diet group member's basic problem was attitude: She didn't rejoice about being rid of undesirable sweet foods; she thought of her abstinence as a "sacrifice." *Sacrifice* is a powerful negative word for overeaters.

Like many overweight people, this woman was defiant, resistant, angry, and frustrated—not a frame of mind conducive to achievement. Joan didn't expect much success, and she didn't have any.

Make a mental list of your goals and expect to attain them. People usually get what they expect. Joan prepared for a binge, and she got one.

Today, expect the best from yourself. You will get the positive things you expect.

*Today's Action Plan: I will replace all mental binge lists with constructive, goal-directed lists.*

**May 24**                        **Chain-Eating**

*Even after I ate until I was sick, I still had an empty, gnawing feeling in the pit of my stomach.*
                                        *—A woman at a diet group*

Like the chain-smoker who lights a cigarette from the

butt of one just smoked, a chain-eater reaches for a second snack while swallowing the first one.

Chain-eaters are not at peace with their bodies. They interpret every body signal as a demand for food, then feel trapped by an insatiable appetite. Every discomfort, every emotion, every empty minute is translated into a physical need for food.

Get to know all your body's moods. Your body doesn't only hunger; it also wants activity, change, and rest. Nourish all your body's real wants. Feed them with your action program.

Today, see that chain-eating is a destructive response to emotions and misread body signals. You must respond only to your body's real hunger to achieve an energized, winning life.

*Today's Action Plan: I will translate boredom and anxiety as a need to get into action. I will feed my positive wants.*

## May 25                          The Three Mess-Keteers

*Things like sugar, salt, and fats simply weren't available to us in any quantity during the period of our genetic development. We can't handle them in more than trace quantities without causing a malfunction in our basic metabolic systems.*

*—Robert Rodale*

Sweets, salty snacks, and saturated fats are three "civilized foods" that can be harmful. Large quantities of them can make a mess of our metabolic systems.

Fat is Food Enemy Number One. You may think you don't have a problem with fats. "I didn't know," said one overeater, "until I had to go on a gall bladder diet, just how addicted to fats I was."

Sugar is Food Enemy Number Two. Sucrose (sugar) becomes glucose in our bodies, overloads our pancreas, and in time causes a kind of endocrine burnout.

Salt is Food Enemy Number Three. It's implicated in the high blood pressure so many overweight people suffer from. Most foods are over-salted in processing, in cooking, and at the table.

Make a decision to eliminate or cut down all three food enemies. Retrain your taste buds to enjoy the more subtle flavors of fresh, whole foods.

Today, choose to enjoy the natural flavors of food.

*Today's Action Plan: I will explore healthy alternatives to fatty, sugary, and salty foods.*

**May 26**                              **Always Go First Class**

*You are what you think, you become what you think, and what you think becomes reality.*

*—Anonymous*

When you think about your life, always be a first-class thinker. The more success you want, the greater you'll have to think. Focus on where you're going, not on where you've been.

From now on, life is opportunity. The only limits are the ones in your own mind. Stretch your mind, and don't be afraid to shoot for the supposedly unattainable. Go straight to first-class goals.

Use a first-class vocabulary, words that promise achievement. Use words that create winning images: *victory, happiness, hope, energy, action.*

Today, buy a first-class ticket to the rest of your life. You can stretch the limits of your thinking to include anything you want.

*Today's Action Plan: I will not sell myself short. I will imagine the greatest opportunity, then I will make it my goal.*

## May 27            You're Greater than You Think

*To believe is to be strong. Doubt cramps energy. Belief is power.*

         —*Frederick W. Robertson*

It's hard to think of yourself as unique and wonderful if your imagination is cramped by self-deprecation. Some overweight people concentrate on self-criticism so much that they can't accept one kind word for themselves, from themselves or others.

If you have trouble thinking kindly about yourself, maybe your arithmetic is backward. Practice addition, and quit subtracting. Instead of devaluing your every act, add value. If you can't believe in your uniqueness, act as if you can. You can't act that way for very long without beginning to like yourself better.

You can win a new image of yourself, a new peace within yourself, a new idea of what life can be. Stretch your mind until you can see your unique worth.

Today, you are heading in the right direction. You will no longer hold yourself back from your own potential by devaluing yourself.

*Today's Action Plan: I will add value to what I do today. I will concentrate on my assets.*

## May 28            No Retreat

*If you get into the habit of retreating from challenges, you're just a sitting duck for regrets.*

         —*Gail Godwin*

All of life challenges you. But how have you met the challenges? Review your life right now. What do you regret most? Probably the challenges you did not meet, the times you said, "I could never do that!"

You said that because you believed it was true. And it was true, because to meet challenges, you need to believe in your own importance.

Whatever your challenge today, believe that you can do it. When you do, your mind and spirit find ingenious ways to accomplish the job. Believing that you already have the solution opens the door to solutions you didn't realize you had.

Today, accept every challenge, believing you can do the job. Having a sense of your own worth opens the door to solutions.

*Today's Action Plan: I won't retreat from any challenge. I will look for can-do solutions.*

**May 29**                    **Cynicism Never Lost a Pound**

*Everything in the world is done by hope.*
*—Martin Luther*

Do you have the will to hope or are you caught in cynicism? "I've tried everything," you say. "Diet, exercise, fad, trend—nothing works for me." You are overwhelming hope with negatives, and without hope there is only cynicism.

If you're lost in destructive, despairing feelings, there is a way to get your hope back. Paraphrase Blaise Pascal's wager about the existence of God. Say, "I've got everything to win if my action plan works, and nothing to lose if it doesn't. So why not go along?"

Hope is positive food for the mind. What your mind consumes today determines habits, attitudes, and capacity to change. The question isn't *whether* you'll change today, but *how*. Hope says the change will be constructive.

Today, you can win by feeding your mind hope. From now on, bet on yourself. It's a sure thing that you're going to win that bet.

*Today's Action Plan: I will drop a loser's cynicism. I will feed my mind the positive food of hope.*

## May 30                    Get Ready, Get Set, Get Motivated

*If it weren't for the group support, I don't think I could make it.*

*—Diet group member*

Support is essential to keep most overeaters going once they're on the road back to winning health. That support can come from one partner or a whole group, as long as you have similar goals and the necessary understanding of a shared experience. No one can help an overeater like another overeater.

Humans are essentially tribal. Most of us enjoy company, but those in trouble really *need* company. If you talk about a particular problem you're having, it helps a great deal when someone in the group simply says, "I know how you feel." Groups perform a valuable function for overeaters—they can help you stay highly motivated.

Today, whether you need a whole group or just another person to confide in, go out and get the support you need.

*Today's Action Plan: I will look for group support for my program.*

*It takes the body twenty-one days to accept new behavior.*

—*Dr. Susan Jones*

Your school reunion is only two weeks away. You climb on the bathroom scale to see how much weight you have to lose to get into your favorite dress—and you panic. Next you set an unrealistic goal, allow yourself too little time, become discouraged, and binge. Then you either stay at home on the big day or wear an old outfit you vowed you would never wear again.

Setting goals is what this book is all about. As the ninth principle of your action plan recommends, take weight loss, exercise, and attitude change in steps. Set small, realistic goals on your way to the big goal.

Give every change in your life—whether it's a food or character change—at least three weeks. This is the time it takes for your body and mind to accept the change as natural.

Today, use this formula to achieve a leaner, more attractive body—allowing sufficient time and setting reachable goals.

*Today's Action Plan: I will set a goal and allow three weeks for change.*

**June 1**                                              **Your Body**

*A body is forsaken when it becomes a source of pain
and humiliation instead of pleasure and pride.*
*—Alexander Lowen*

Your greatest task today is to create the best possible
environment to promote healthy weight loss. To do
this, you must move away from a pervasive sense of
body-hate.

Your body's appearance is the result of a lifetime of
choices. When you make different choices, you change
your body. Making changes is sometimes painful, but it
can be either the hopeless pain of staying an overeater
or the joyful pain of changing what, how, and why you
eat. You can choose to change.

Make the right eating choices beginning today, and
the negative way you feel about your body will begin to
disappear. You'll feel comfortable within yourself.

Today, end a painful estrangement from your body.
From now on, your body will reflect your good food
and exercise choices.

*Today's Action Plan: I will make a commitment to
befriend my body.*

*Many of us die with our music unplayed.*
—*Mary Kay Ash*

Two conflicting voices carry on constant tune-playing in your head. One chants, "Help me!" The other sings, "Don't be a crybaby." Because these voices don't harmonize, we tend to ignore both when we should heed both.

It takes courage to ask sincerely for help from our family, a supportive friend, doctor, or diet group. It takes courage to stand firm and battle your food problem.

Find the hero within you. This hero may reach out to others with an eating problem, or this hero may summon the strength and knowledge within to change. Either way, your theme song is played without a sour note.

Prepare for success. When you believe you are a hero, so you will act like a hero.

Today, hear the voices searching for the hero in you. When you listen to life's music, it will be *your* song.

*Today's Action Plan: I will find the hero in myself. I will have the courage to either seek help or take an individual stand.*

*An excuse is worse and more terrible than a lie; for an excuse is a lie guarded.*
—*Alexander Pope*

"Both my parents are overweight." "There's been a recent death in my family." "I have too many money worries." "Nobody likes me." Are these good excuses to overeat?

A good excuse is a powerful enemy of weight-goal achievement. You may come from an overweight family, you may have suffered a terrible pain lately, you may be seriously short of funds, or your social life may be depressing. But the more often you repeat your excuse, the more convinced you are that it is true.

Throw away the notion that if only this problem would disappear, you would be able to control your overeating.

Today, see that all excuses, good and bad, are damaging. Make a yes decision to get rid of all excuses to overeat.

*Today's Action Plan: I will get rid of all my excuses. I will be fully in charge.*

## June 4                                                    Anger

*Anger is only one letter short of danger.*
                                              *—Anonymous*

The overeater's personality is often defined as angry. No wonder—we overeaters are labeled, libeled, and laughed at! But even justified anger is dangerous to an overeater. We don't get even when we eat, only fat.

Successful people encounter embarrassing, depressing situations too. But they choose to dwell on positive memories, not unpleasantness, and let go of destructive experiences. Unsuccessful people dwell on the situation until they make it a concrete memory they can't free their minds of.

Strange as it seems, the most important thing in your life today isn't to lose weight. It is to become a person who doesn't hoard anger and handle difficulties with a knife and fork. Weight loss will follow.

Today, learn to handle anger as an achiever. You have seen how anger easily spells danger.

*Today's Action Plan: I will not eat as a solution to unpleasantness. I will practice making positive memories.*

## June 5                                    Not Strictly from Hunger

*Everything agitates me, and I experience every agitation as a sensation of hunger, even if I have just eaten.*
— Ellen West

We overeaters eat with our mouths and our feelings. Every situation and every emotion, negative and positive, cues us to eat. Food has become our reaction to every stimulus.

If we eat in response to everything, what happens when our body sends us true hunger messages? We don't recognize them. We have to learn to discern real hunger from emotional hunger.

When you are following a weight-losing plan and your body suddenly says, "Feed me now," look for the cause of the hunger. If you determine it's emotional hunger, work on the emotion. If it's real hunger, get busy and wait for the next planned meal.

Today, recognize the difference between emotional and physical hunger. You will begin to teach your hunger patience.

*Today's Action Plan: I will not eat because of an emotion. I will lose pounds and gain patience.*

*When you insist you're not the kind of person who can climb a mountain or make a speech, all you are saying is that up to now you haven't done it.*
> —Mildred Newman
> Bernard Berkowitz

You give yourself a lot of attention—negative attention. Every day you tell yourself that you are the "most awful," "stupidest," "fattest" person in the world. You sell yourself short with such self-deprecation. It shows through in everything you do. Make peace with yourself!

Start paying some positive attention to yourself. What are your fine points? You want to change, you have the courage to face yourself, and you have the commitment to work for greater self-understanding. People who take this action are not "awful," "stupid," or "fat."

You are a creator of solutions. You are giving yourself this chance today. Aim for the top of a problem and start climbing.

Today, refuse to pay only negative attention to yourself. It is finally time to be as fair to yourself as you are to others.

*Today's Action Plan: I will not deprecate anything I am or do. I will pay only positive attention to myself.*

*Instead of crying over spilt milk, go milk another cow.*
> —Anonymous

The quotation above is an action version of "Don't cry over spilt milk," only it goes one important step further. We must *do* something about a problem, not just lie down and accept it.

You are one who converts every problem into an opportunity. You must be, or else you'd be waiting for luck instead of reading this book. The door to a winning future is open to you.

Remind yourself every day that you are far better than you think you are. You know you want to attain a healthy weight, and you're learning how to do that. You have a mind fully equipped to work out your problems. You are a creator of solutions.

You are doing so many things right. Today, remind yourself that you are a better person than you ever thought you were.

*Today's Action Plan: When problems arise, I will not simply cry. I will go one important step further; I will get into action to create new solutions.*

**June 8**                                         **Positive Concentration**

*Believe that life is worth living, and your belief will create the fact.*

*—William James*

Concentrate on the positive events of today. Your mind will readily cast aside old, negative memories if you cooperate.

Think back to the pleasant memories of your childhood, school days, your first job. Look at some favorite old pictures. You tend to remember the happy times you had.

Your mind has a tendency to shrivel unpleasant memories and give back a generalized rosy glow. This is your mind's way of protecting you from the pain that negative memories can inflict. Your mind wants to cancel destructive ego experiences. Why don't you let it?

Today, see how your mind rejects unpleasant

memories. Letting go of unpleasant memories is possible when you consciously remember happiness.

*Today's Action Plan: I will reject the negative. I will concentrate on the positive.*

## June 9                                              Conscience Power

*Every worthwhile accomplishment, big or little, has its stages of drudgery and triumph; a beginning, a struggle, and a victory.*

*—Anonymous*

The second principle in your action plan advises you to practice confidence every day. One of the best ways to do this is to keep your conscience clean. The power of your conscience is enormous. It can lead you straight to your inevitable victory over destructive eating.

Harness the power of your conscience by doing what you know is right for you—following your eating plan and exercising for weight loss. Your self-confidence will grow and you will free yourself of guilt, which erodes self-confidence. When you gain confidence, other people will reflect confidence back to you.

Today, mobilize the power of your conscience to build confidence. Rid yourself of guilt by doing what is right for you.

*Today's Action Plan: I will keep my conscience clean and powerful.*

## June 10                                          Exercise Should Be Fun

*I discovered aerobic dancing, something I really enjoyed. What a difference it has made in my weight and health!*

*—A woman at a diet group*

Often, we assume that if exercise is good for us, we won't like it. Do you believe exercise needs to hurt and be unpleasant if it is to work?

You should love the exercise you do. Of course, you'll love the results—an energized body, sharp mind, vented frustrations, and burned-off fat. But the best way to get these results is for exercise to be fun. Unless it's fun, only a few utterly determined people can stick with it long enough to be rewarded.

Create positive exercise experiences, ones you will look forward to every day. Try everything—aerobic dance, swimming, jogging, bicycling, walking, or any combination of these. Which exercise do you love?

Today, make exercise one of the most enjoyable experiences of your day.

*Today's Action Plan: I will discover the exercises that are most fun for me to do. I will do them.*

## June 11          A New Way to Climb Off that Plateau

*I hit a weight plateau, got discouraged, and slipped off the program. I felt as if I just couldn't cut my calories any lower.*

*—A diet group member*

While losing weight, there comes a time when the body temporarily stops losing pounds. You're still doing what you should, yet your eating and exercise plan no longer seems to work. A weight plateau can be discouraging enough to send us back to overeating.

The usual advice to people on plateaus is to wait it out until you start losing again or cut your caloric intake even more. But why not double your exercise instead? If you are exercising twenty minutes a day, exercise forty minutes. By increasing your oxygen delivery rate, your body will begin to burn fat more efficiently. Not only will you begin to lose weight again, but you'll improve strength and flexibility, which makes it easier for you to exercise. See what a marvelous cycle you can create?

Today, instead of giving up, try a new solution for beating the plateau blahs.

*Today's Action Plan: I will create an exercise solution for the plateau problem. I will increase my exercise time.*

### June 12                                    Do You Wanna Dance?

*I love to dance, but my husband doesn't. Dance aerobics is the perfect exercise for me.*
*—Overheard at dance exercise class*

Exercise can fill more than one empty spot in your life. If you want to dance but you don't have Fred Astaire or Ginger Rogers for a partner, a dance class can be your personal exercise and fulfill your dancing fantasy as well. Again, the point is to find an exercise that you like.

The benefits will increase too. If you exercise for more than forty minutes at a strenuous pace, your body releases natural opiates, called endorphins, which give you a tremendous lift.

Today you're on the exercise fast track. You have a deeper sense of security, knowing that you have the stamina and strength to do anything you want.

*Today's Action Plan: I will make fitness my top priority. I will choose exercise for a partner in life.*

*Enthusiasm: It is nothing more nor less than faith in action.*

—*Henry Chester*

The tour bus traveled across the bleak, treeless Outer Hebrides landscape. All the sightseers were bored but one. "This is fantastic," the woman repeated, as she snapped pictures of scrubby fields of heather. Her fellow passengers stared unbelievingly. The woman was obviously enjoying herself. But how?

At the end of the bus ride, a curious passenger approached "Mrs. Fantastic," as she became known. "Thank you for making the trip more enjoyable for everyone," he said. "But don't tell me you really enjoyed that ride!" Smiling, she answered, "I certainly did. I learned something long ago in the theater. A good actress doesn't just play a part, she lives it." Her eyes twinkled. "You see, my act still works."

Today, be an enthusiastic person, an actor if necessary. You will develop enthusiasm in others, which comes right back to you.

*Today's Action Plan: I will be enthusiastic wherever I am, whatever I do. I will be a good-news person.*

## June 14                          What Do You Want from Food?

*Keep no secrets of thyself from thyself.*

—*Greek proverb*

Plato said that the unexamined life is not worth living. But overweight people avoid one particular examination: What do we find in food? We overeat because of feelings, as if food held answers to our human loneliness. We turn to food when we need companionship, comfort, reassurance, or a sense of well-being.

Examine how you use food. Some people overeat to quiet emotional need. But what cookie gives you affection? What piece of cake hugs you? What chocolate bar whispers, "I love you"?

Food can't replace human contact. Another person may not return the love or friendship you offer, but it's a risk worth taking. Human relationships may not always work out, but they won't add to your weight problem.

Today, face the question "What do I want from food?" Food cannot give you the emotional support that will help you be thin.

*Today's Action Plan: I will examine how I used food. I will not try to satisfy my emotions with food.*

## June 15              Success Enemy Number One

*Fear is the darkroom where negatives are developed.*
*—Anonymous*

The survival fears that pumped adrenaline into the veins of our ancestors are gone. Today's everyday fears of failure, embarrassment, and loneliness are likely to be based on emotional rather than physical survival. Whatever its roots, fear stops you from grasping at opportunities. It tricks you into thinking your physical letdown after an adrenaline rush is hunger.

Fear, manifested in anxiety or panic or worry, can mean you lack confidence in yourself. But you can develop confidence by getting into action. If you fear doing something, do it; otherwise, you avoid it with one binge after another.

Fear saps energy and increases hunger feelings. Today, decide to get the action habit and defeat your fears.

*Today's Action Plan: I will not attempt to solve fear by overeating. I will face each fear with its action solution.*

## June 16                                    Don't Resign Yourself to Fat

*If we want a thing badly enough, we can make it happen. If we let ourselves be discouraged, that is proof that our wanting was inadequate.*
—*Dorothy L. Sayers*

Have you ever thought, "I'll just have to learn to live with this weight. Mature, intelligent people accept the inevitable."

Don't resign yourself to a fat life. Don't accept being depressed and feeling second-rate because of your weight. You deserve the best, so get into action. Want to fulfill your desires. Want life to deliver good things. Want success. These are all winners' wants.

Defeat disbelief by believing you can achieve whatever you want. Use your intelligence by putting your desires into action. Having this book in your hands this minute is a good start. You are determined to keep your desire for a high-energy life at peak level.

Today, choose never to resign yourself to an unhappy, unproductive, immobilized life.

*Today's Action Plan: I will think myself worthy of my greatest desires. I will act rather than resign myself.*

## June 17                                             You're All Right

*The important thing is not where you were or where you are, but where you want to get.*
—*Dave Mahoney*

The first principle in your action plan says you have

a unique worth. If you don't receive praise, don't get a raise, don't attract the lover you want, there's nothing wrong with you. You are still uniquely worthy, and you are not dependent on outside acceptance for your sense of personal value.

Sometimes we give other people permission to criticize us. Don't play that game. You are the sum total of your own choices. You are responsible, not dependent. When one of your choices proves to be negative, you see clearly what needs to be done and you do it.

Your "all rightness" does not need validation from anyone but you. Today, develop a solid understanding of your unique worth.

*Today's Action Plan: I will be all right no matter what happens. I will be responsible, never apologizing, for my life.*

## June 18        The 10 Percent Solution

*The less one has to do, the less time one finds to do it in.*

—*Lord Chesterfield*

Busy people seem to know how to organize their time and always seem to be able to take on just a little bit more. You can be that kind of person. Increase whatever you do by 10 percent, and soon you'll have a deserved reputation as a doer.

There isn't one thing you are doing in your life right now that you couldn't do better. You could increase your exercise time by 10 percent. That may seem like a trifle, but it adds up to something significant over a week, month, or year.

Instead of strolling down the street, walk 10 percent faster. You get more exercise, you arrive earlier, and you feel more determined. Wouldn't you like to push against the old limits? Ten percent more—that's all.

Today, ask 10 percent more of yourself. It's a good feeling to know you can accomplish that.

*Today's Action Plan: I will become 10 percent better at everything I do.*

**June 19**                                              **Stress Solution**

*Most of today's stress problems require a behavioral solution, not a physical one.*
                                            *—Dr. Herbert Benson*

Most of us lead a pressure-cooker existence. Traffic jams, job anxiety, and odd responsibilities all combine to jangle our nerves and tense our muscles. Too often an overweight person's answer to stress is overeating, a physical response instead of a simple behavior change.

Remember the last time you were really stressed? Your breathing was rapid and shallow. This time, apply the brakes. Begin a seven-second breathe-in, breathe-out cycle. Repeat this eight times, and in about two minutes, stress is gone.

By responding to stress this way, you won't be heaping overeating stress on top of what you already have. Try this small change in behavior anywhere, anytime.

Today, you learned a behavioral solution for everyday stress. You see that there are constructive ways to solve problems, which means you never need to turn to overeating again.

*Today's Action Plan: I will seek nonfood solutions to life's stresses.*

> *My duty, as an intellectual, is to think, to think without restriction, even at the risk of blundering. I must set no limits within myself, and I must let no limits be set for me.*
> *—Jean Paul Sartre*

Dream no small dreams. Small dreams limit your imagination. Great dreams recognize no limits—including the limitation of excess weight.

Your new life—the life of controlled eating, exercise, and take-charge attitudes—is not a struggle, but a cooperation with yourself. Overeating used to bring you into conflict with your own intelligence, triggering struggle and self-disgust. Those days are gone forever.

Great dreamers set no inner limits and recognize no outer limits. They know that the harder they go, the closer they come to achievement.

Today, prepare yourself to dream great dreams and to put them into action quickly. You are a mover, unlimited and undaunted.

> *Today's Action Plan: I will allow no limits within or without myself. I will get into action and cooperate with life.*

> *"After a long day at work, I don't have the energy to exercise." "I get enough exercise around the house." "Exercising only makes me hungrier."*
> *—Results of Harris Poll*

Exercise is one key to permanent weight loss. So if you're not exercising, you must have a good excuse. Is it one of the three offered by polled adults who don't exercise?

"After a long day on the job, I don't have any energy left." Wrong! When you're de-energized, you need to exercise most. Remain inactive, and you spend your evening exhausted. Exercise creates energy!

"I get enough exercise around the house/job/school." Wrong again! You may work hard, stopping and starting dozens of time, but few jobs give you the sustained aerobic exercise you need for your health.

"Exercise makes me hungrier." Still wrong! Exercise is an appetite suppressant. You'll eat less after you exercise, and your body will burn more calories.

Find three good reasons to exercise instead: "I'll burn more calories." "I'll feel better." "I'll look better."

Today, you heard three bad excuses not to exercise and saw right through them. You found three smart reasons to exercise instead.

*Today's Action Plan: I will be fit. I will treat my body like a muscle born to be worked.*

## June 22                                          Dr. Right

*Doctors have laughed at me, scolded me, and refused to treat me if I didn't lose weight.*
                              *—Overheard at a diet club*

At a diet group meeting, one woman said, "No matter what I go to the doctor for, he blames it on my weight." Another woman added, "I've been humiliated so many times that I don't go to my doctor even when I should."

You have a right to the best medical care available. If any doctor treats you in less than a dignified manner, fire him or her. You may very well want your doctor to guide you on certain parts of your weight program, but that's your decision to make or to change anytime you wish.

If you're unhappy with your present physician, find another. Doctor Right will be supportive of your efforts, will be optimistic about your new program, and will never bully you.

Today, and from now on, expect dignified and attentive service from your physician and the medical staff.

*Today's Action Plan: I will respect myself and demand the same from the professionals I pay. I will have the medical help I need and deserve.*

## June 23                    Become a Now Person

*It is vain to say human beings ought to be satisfied with tranquillity; they must have action, and they will make it if they cannot find it.*

—*Charlotte Brontë*

When you postpone weight-losing action with "tomorrow" promises, you are implying that conditions will be better at some special future time. But when that time arrives, conditions usually aren't. Now is all you ever have to use, whatever the conditions.

Be a doer, not a procrastinator; an optimist, not a pessimist. You know what you want your life to be. If you don't like your life, you can change it.

You are perfectly capable of putting together the best program for your life, capable of achieving it, and capable of living with your achievement. Success is an idea you can act on.

Today be satisfied with nothing less than action. You have the capacity to become a doer and an optimist.

*Today's Action Plan: I will make today's conditions just right for action. And I'll start now.*

*The spirit that does not soar is destined to grovel.*
                                    *—Benjamin Disraeli*

The world is moving. The way to keep pace with it is to set goals, not just make wishes. "I'm going to lose X number of pounds, get down to my natural weight, become physically fit, and win success in my life." Goals such as these give you a definite idea of where you want to go.

Ten years seems like a long time, but before you know it, it will pass. Where do you want to be ten years from today? What do you want to accomplish on the job, at home, in your social life? What do you want to look like? Write it down. This is your plan of action.

To make this ten-year plan a reality, begin to set smaller goals. Each small goal achieved is a step toward winning.

Today, look at the next decade and take charge of where you want to be.

*Today's Action Plan: I will soar into the rest of my life by making a ten-year plan and setting the goals to achieve it.*

*Our deeds determine us, as much as we determine our deeds.*

                                    *—George Eliot*

What does the word *success* mean to you? It means controlled eating, a fit body, and a take-charge attitude. Those are fantastic goals, worthy of you.

But don't expect perfection from yourself or your life. Expect that you will continue to change; be open to it. Expect that others will not be able to fulfill you; fulfill yourself. Expect that others will not be responsible for you; own yourself.

As you grow in confidence, you will feel more and more that you have embarked on a rewarding relationship with yourself. As the months pass, it will evolve into a caring, trusting companionship based on self-regard and winning attitudes.

Today, evaluate your performance and reaffirm your resolve to take charge of the food in your life.

*Today's Action Plan: I will renew my commitment to success. Today I will move one small goal closer to my desired body.*

## June 26                This Is the Day

*Seize this day! Begin now! Each day is a new life. Seize it. Live it. For in today already walks tomorrow.*
*—David Guy Powers*

Isn't it amazing how we take the numbers on the calendar for granted? Each day is a miracle waiting to happen to you.

This day you will not accept the number 26 on the calendar as just another mark on paper. Today will be a day that will leave a mark on your life. Each day marks a move toward a life of achievement, a life of victory over food.

Today is the most precious of your possessions. No one can take it from you. It can be thrown away, but it is unstealable. Use the wonderful gift of today.

Of all the right things you have done today, the most right is your commitment to make this day, and each day of your life, well-lived.

*Today's Action Plan: I will seize this day. I will make this day count in some special way.*

*In the supermarket, a little boy said in a loud voice, "Mommy, what makes people fat?" I didn't turn around; I knew he was pointing at me.*
        *—A diet group member*

Does criticism from others throw you into a defensive mode? The only cure for this is to be safe in the knowledge of the changes you're making. You know who you are and where you're going. Soon others will see and know it too.

You don't have to own cruel remarks based on your size. And don't feel that every mention of weight is aimed at you.

When you are accomplishing what you know you want to accomplish, your mind is at peace. Your mind is positive and is drawn to the positive. You may overhear negative things, but they don't belong to you.

Today, be too self-respectful to take any abusive remarks seriously. Your new positive outlook will attract constructive comment and shed the negative.

*Today's Action Plan: I will disown any cruel remarks based on my size. I will concentrate on maintaining the positive attitude that will bring me a thinner, healthier body and a happier life.*

*Everything comes to him who hustles while he waits.*
        *—Thomas A. Edison*

Pressure, from outside and inside, is a part of our times. We try to do our very best, hoping others will take notice and be pleased. Business people strive for that big promotion. Children take school exams and worry that they may not pass.

The important thing in any pressure situation is not to overeat while awaiting the outcome. Successful authors learn that once they mail a precious manuscript to a publisher, they must hustle right on to a new book. If a rejection notice comes, they're so immersed in the new project that the turndown doesn't hurt nearly as much.

Hustle while you wait. If you sit around expectantly waiting for praise, you'll be crushed if you don't get it. But if you've moved on to something new and interesting, you're not apt to get bogged down in self-pity.

Today, make accomplishing the job the most important thing. Then get going on the next job.

*Today's Action Plan: I won't lock my life into a holding pattern during a pressure situation. I will do my job and then hustle on.*

## June 29                                       Pressure Well-Met

*As exercise strengthens the body, pressure well-met strengthens the spirit.*

—*Ira Wolff*

When you're under pressure—starting a new job, moving to a new home, any major life change—don't use food as a safety valve. Overeating only gives the illusion of control while it ravages your self-esteem, leaving your body and mind weaker. When pressure builds, there is no better release than physical exercise. Your mind is distracted when your body is engaged.

Pressure well-met, whether by exercise or attitude, simply means pressure well-used. Wherever there is pressure, there is a challenge. Pressure is essential to winners; it's the kick in the pants that helps them get to the top. Pressure causes you to concentrate your energy completely.

Today your safety valve for pressure comes from healthy eating, exercise, and your new take-charge attitude. Concentrate on these and win.

*Today's Action Plan: I will use pressure to help me concentrate on my goals. I will concentrate on winning.*

## June 30                    What's to Become of You?

*You will become as small as your controlling desire, as great as your dominant aspiration.*
                                            —*James Allen*

Suppose you're faced with hiring one of two people: the first has great talent, but is a pessimist; the second has average ability, but bubbles with enthusiasm. You'd do well to employ the second person—enthusiasm gets the job done. Enthusiasm gives birth to endurance, whereas pessimism kills it.

You have one great aspiration: to take charge of each day to shake your food dependency. Overeating made your life a muddle. Now you've rejected excess food as a way to manage your life.

Keep your mind on achieving a thinner winner's life; stay too busy to be unsure. Look for the best within you, and keep finding it. Enthusiasm is belief that caught fire!

Today, see that enthusiasm fired by belief in yourself will help you reach your life goal. You are becoming the kind of person everyone admires.

*Today's Action Plan: I will pursue my goals enthusiastically. I will work my action plan persistently.*

JULY

**July 1**                                       **A Small Beginning**

*It matters not how small the beginning may seem to be; what is once well done is done forever.*
*—Henry David Thoreau*

We all have basic wants: security, health, comfort, confidence, admiration, and self-improvement. Overeating strikes at every one of these basic desires. Is it any wonder your overeating produces such anxiety?

The most important thing for you to do is to make a beginning, right now, no matter how overweight you are. You may think there is no hope for you. Banish such thoughts from your mind! Today your heart will beat 103,680 times, you'll breathe 23,040 times, and you'll speak 4,800 words. Make every beat, breath, and word count as a beginning toward your winning life.

Today, open your mind to a new way to achieve your basic needs.

*Today's Action Plan: I will make a small beginning by improving my weight-loss plan. With every heartbeat, breath, and word, I will make today work.*

**July 2**                                      **Overcoming Despair**

*The darkest hour is only sixty minutes.*
*—Anonymous*

If you've overeaten, you probably feel lethargic,

headachy, hungover. Emotionally, you feel ashamed, disgusted, despairing. Overeating was your attempt to make life more comfortable, but you need a better coping solution than that.

"Imagineering" is a way to overcome the despair of the overeating trap. Try picturing the person you want to become, then dream his or her dream. Visualize the healthy, attractive body within your present body. Dwell on this vision.

Today, your darkest hour of overeating can be changed to a bright new idea of self-imagining. You can achieve what you want by dreaming a greater dream, and then seeing yourself in it.

*Today's Action Plan: I will see overeating as an act that doesn't work. Instead, I will imagine my body as I want it to be.*

## July 3                                      Get the Review Habit

*There is only one success—to be able to spend your life in your own way.*
*—Christopher Morley*

This month, you'll be reviewing the principles of your action plan. As with anything you really want to learn, you must review and repeat these principles until you make them as much a habit as your old destructive behavior. Repeat positive actions often enough, and you will create new habits and erase bad ones.

Life is meant to be a glorious adventure. As you put your thinking into action, life can also be a marvelous challenge. And as long as you are working your action plan, you are not overeating. You can't raise your self-esteem and do what you despise at the same time.

You are worthy of your love and care. This month, use review to know yourself better and to grow in self-love. If you do, you can begin to live life your own way.

Today, begin to review and repeat the principles of your action plan until you make them part of you.

*Today's Action Plan: I will review the principles of my plan until they are part of me. I will grow in self-worth.*

## July 4 — Your Unique Worth

*All mental and spiritual health begins with self-acceptance.*
*—Samuel Butler*

Some discouraged overeaters find it difficult to believe they are worthy people. Yet to achieve the weight loss they seek, they must achieve self-acceptance—a supreme consciousness of self-worth. That is why principle number one says, "Develop a solid understanding of your unique worth."

Perhaps you said, "I want to, but . . ." You added *but* because you felt helpless. You believed you were too weak to take action to get out of a rut. You were wrong.

*Want* to save yourself enough to make your action plan work for you. Make such a want your action for today. Positive action halts any lurking "I can'ts."

Today, accept the idea of your unique worth and build greater confidence and strength by getting into action.

*Today's Action Plan: I will stop the flow of "I can'ts." I will accept and understand my unique worth.*

## July 5 — Imagineering

*When the will and the imagination are antagonistic, it is always the imagination which wins, without any exception.*
*—Émile Coué*

If you concentrate all the sun's energy through a magnifying glass onto a pile of twigs, you'll start a fire. Likewise, if you can concentrate your imagination on one goal, you will ignite your wishes into a flame of action. The secret is to concentrate all your imagination on what you want most.

Imagine the body you want, the one that already exists within you. Concentrate all your imaginative power on it. Your concentrated imagination is infinitely more powerful than when it is scattered among a long list of wants.

"Imagineering" is simply giving a pictured form to your goal. It is a powerful way of giving substance to your wishes and thereby making them happen.

Today, focus all your imaginative energy on one desire, the look and feel of your new body.

*Today's Action Plan: I will concentrate all my imagination on my beautiful inner body to make it visible. I will be an imaginative doer.*

## July 6            Practice Confidence

*Keep on doing what it took to get started.*
*—John L. McCaffrey*

The second principle in your plan says, "Practice confidence every day." Can you actually develop confidence in yourself by practicing it? You bet you can. And with an emerging confidence in yourself, you will whip your weight problem.

Indecision saps your emotional strength. It laughs at your goals and tangles you in confusion. Confidence, on the other hand, expects—even demands—that you achieve and win.

Nothing builds your confidence faster than achieving

small goals right away and every day. So get into action. Make your goal for today eating right for eventual weight loss. Losing weight is important, but even more important is achieving the smaller goal of healthy eating for one day. What a confidence builder!

Indecision is the killer of dreams. Today, replace indecision with a thinning, winning confidence.

*Today's Action Plan: I will practice confidence by achieving a minimum of one small goal a day.*

### July 7                                  You Have a Good Thing

*He that labors in any great or laudable undertaking has his fatigues first supported by hope and afterward rewarded by joy.*

—*Dr. Samuel Johnson*

You've heard the old saying "Where there is life, there is hope." Actually that's backward. Where there is *hope,* there is *life.* There is no life without hope. When you read these pages, you prove that you are hopeful and very much alive.

Hope helps you imagine how it will feel when you look in the mirror and see your new, vibrant, attractive body. Hope helps you dream, set, and reach goals.

Hope is an essential part of the good beginning you make every day. It will lift you out of the overeater's shadow of despair into the sunshine of the winner's circle. Hope cancels out despair.

Today, trade your shackled existence for a life filled with hope. Hope and action will lead straight to joyous living.

*Today's Action Plan: I will put hope first so that I can live. I will take action and do what I want most in this world.*

*Nothing is a greater impediment to being on good*
*terms with others than being ill at ease with yourself.*
                                    —*Honoré de Balzac*

The third action principle says, "Radiate warmth."
Your caring warmth should flow in two directions: out
to others and in to your deepest self. Being overweight
in a thin-is-right society is enough of a burden, but suffering without warmth and self-caring is downright
unbearable. And you must give warmth first—especially to yourself—before you can receive it.

Loving yourself just as you are today, however imperfect, is like turning on an x ray that reveals the real you
underneath the flesh. Self-love not only gives you the
capacity to care about others, it also gives you the
strength and confidence to make changes in your life.

Today, judge yourself with a caring heart. You create
the darkness in your life when you stand in the way of
your own light.

*Today's Action Plan: I will radiate caring without and*
*within.*

*Happiness is the exercise of vital powers, along lines of*
*excellence, in a life affording them scope.*
                                    —*Edith Hamilton*

Your life needs a focal point to give it meaning. A life
filled with aimless rounds of meaningless activities dis-
sipates your vital powers. It tires and bores you. For an
overeater, lacking a goal is a catastrophe; food binges are
inevitable in an attempt to overcome the emptiness.

Every day, you uncover talents and strive for excellence.

Make today count. The most satisfying way an overeater can do this is to eat and exercise for physical and mental fitness. Concentrate all your powers on this point.

Today you'll accomplish things because of your positive thoughts. Put the positive side of your mind to work. It's right for you.

Today, develop the right focus, and use all your power to reach it.

*Today's Action Plan: I will focus all my energy on my ultimate weight goal. I trust that what I think will work for me.*

## July 10 Fears

*You may not realize it when it happens, but a kick in the teeth may be the best thing in the world for you.*
—*Walt Disney*

Principle number four in your plan says, "Learn what your fears are." Fear hides behind many disguises. The biggest fear you mask is that you will not be able to withstand a kick in the teeth. No matter how many times you fight back from defeat, a negative critic inside you insists that you are doomed to fail.

When we overeaters don't recognize past courage, we're practicing a negative arithmetic. We may have overcome adversity ten times in the past year. But if only once we didn't, our negative critic subtracts one from ten and gets zero.

Fear is a lack of confidence in our future behavior, and the only antidote for that is action. Fear tells you to quit; self-confidence tells you that when you fight your way through fear you can't fail, because even if you lose, you learn. Then you can go on to win next time.

Today, make courage count more than fear of failing. Since you learn from every mistake, there is no such thing as failing.

*Today's Action Plan: I will subtract one from ten and get confidence.*

## July 11                                     Be All Here

*We can be completely present. We can be all here. We can give all our attention to the opportunity before us.*
*—Mark Van Doren*

Give all your attention to the opportunity of this day. Be all here. Be completely in the now. Above all, want to be with yourself today.

We try to wiggle out and escape from the present for just one reason: to be rid of ourselves. What folly! Self-hate is spiritually unconstitutional. It's a cruelty that breaks the laws of love and humanity.

Today, do what you know you want to do, become a little more of what you want to be, and gracefully move your body, mind, and spirit further from the desire for excess food.

See today as a great opportunity to be really present for yourself, to be all here for you. Banish from this day of opportunity any imagined need to overeat.

*Today's Action Plan: I will be all here. Whatever opportunity this day holds, I will seize it.*

## July 12                                   Burning Desire

*The dream of yesterday is the hope of today and the reality of tomorrow.*
*—Robert H. Goddard*

The fifth principle in your action plan says, "Acknowledge a burning desire to be thin and healthy." The key is the word *acknowledge*. Overeat, and your unacknowledged desire is drowned by food. But acknowledge your desire to yourself, even to the world, and it becomes so strong that it refuses to be suppressed.

Acknowledge your resolve that today you will not overeat. You will do exactly what you want to do. If you act on your desires, you can't do what you despise.

What is tomorrow's reality? It's freedom from excess food and unwanted flesh. It's being creative, energized, and physically and mentally fit. All this, because today you have a burning desire to be thin and healthy.

To suppress this burning desire is to risk smothering it with extra food. Today, you won't take that risk.

*Today's Action Plan: I will acknowledge, to myself and others, that I have a powerful desire to be thin and healthy.*

**July 13**                                    **Get in the Game!**

*My friends thought I was crazy—tennis at my age and weight!*

*—Woman at a tournament*

Is there an exercise or sport that interests you, but you're too embarrassed to try it? "I was forty-nine years old and weighed 185 pounds when we moved to our new condo with tennis courts," said one woman. "For several weeks, I stared at those courts wishing I was twenty-five and thin.

"One day," she went on, "I ran into the resident pro. To make conversation, I said, 'I'd be one of your pupils if only I were twenty years younger and many pounds lighter.' Ignoring my excuse, the pro offered me a complimentary lesson."

Five years later, this woman weighed only 135 pounds and played tournament tennis. "It wasn't easy to get out there," she said, "but I forced myself, and I'm happy I did. Now I feel stronger—both physically and emotionally."

Today, reconsider the sports and exercises that you have been too timid to try.

*Today's Action Plan: From this day on, I will not limit my exercise horizons. I will move more today than ever before—and keep moving.*

### July 14                                    Your Own Sunlight

*It is the artist's business to create sunshine when the sun fails.*

—*Romain Rolland*

You are the artist of your environment. When it rains on you, you don't have to wait for others to change the landscape. As the sixth principle in your plan says, "Make your own sunlight." You light your own way just as you cast your own dark shadows.

Even the happiest people have some darkness, but the life of overeaters seems especially somber. Self-loathing darkens their way. Doing what you want for yourself can brighten your way.

This principle leads you in one direction: toward healthy eating, physical and mental fitness, a thinner body, and a life of inner comfort. You instinctively know that such a life will light up your environment. The light of action banishes the darkness of depression.

Like an artist, you control the light in your life. Today, by doing for yourself what you know you should, you paint a life with bright colors.

*Today's Action Plan: I will paint my day from the bright colors on my palette. I will light my own way with good choices.*

*Doubt of any kind cannot be resolved except by action.*
*—Thomas Carlyle*

Too many overeaters are immersed in self-awareness, mistakenly believing that learning about themselves is action in itself. But such self-discoveries give us no more than a minor boost unless we use them to take *effective* charge of our lives.

The dictionary defines *effective* as "producing the desired result." Is the way you're living now producing the result you desire?

Today, go beyond feelings and doubts. Your desire to be physically and emotionally fit will power your courage to act. You will eat right, exercise, and get beyond feelings into action. You choose to take effective charge of your life.

Today, when you take effective action, you will produce the results you want—a healthy, winning life.

*Today's Action Plan: I will take effective charge of my life to achieve independence from food.*

*We must have courage to bet on our ideas, to take the calculated risk, and to act. Everyday living requires courage if life is to bring happiness.*
*—Maxwell Maltz*

"Take charge of your life," reads the seventh principle of your action plan. The spice of life, contrary to the popular expression, is not variety; it's choice. And the spiciest, most successful life results from choices well made. Right or wrong, the choices that really work for you are the ones you make for yourself.

This seems so clear, yet many people see themselves as powerless over their own lives. They wait for someone to tell them what to do next.

Success favors active, take-charge people—those who have the courage to take risks and act on their own desires. Bet on yourself as a thin and healthy person today.

Today, take the initiative to get where you want to go. That's the best decision you could make this or any other day.

*Today's Action Plan: I will take charge and make choices that take me closer to independence from overeating.*

## July 17                    A Magnificent Obsession

*The spending of our energies it the greatest possible stimulus to their recreation.*
                                   *—Charles Darwin*

Ray, an overweight, middle-aged business executive, had all the trademarks of a compulsive personality. He was a chain-smoker, a workaholic, and he had a drinking problem as well.

Ray's doctor told him what he already knew, that he was literally killing himself. The doctor urged him to quit overeating, smoking, and drinking, and to try regular exercise.

Shaken by the doctor's dire warnings, Ray followed her instructions. Exercising was tough at first. After jogging a few steps he was gasping and his muscles ached. But eventually he came to love it.

Ray's new love became an obsession. One mile increased to two, then to five. Ray harnessed his compulsiveness into a healthy activity. Can you channel your energies into a beneficial habit as he did?

Today, turn your compulsiveness to your own advantage.

*Today's Action Plan: I will look for an exercise to get healthfully compulsive about. This habit will move me closer to my goal.*

## July 18                                          Do It Now

*Do not look back. It will neither give you back the past nor satisfy your daydreams. Your duty, your reward, your destiny are here and now.*
                                    —*Dag Hammarskjöld*

Today is not just "the first day of the rest of your life"; it's more urgent. It's the only time you have to work with, so, as the eighth principle in your action plan says, "Do whatever needs to be done now." It's quite specific—do what you know you must do.

Deliberately let go of unpleasant overeating memories. If you look back and find failure, regret, or self-deprecation following you, let those feelings go.

Today, move toward the vitally interesting life you want. You aren't limited by yesterday. Today is fresh, joyful, creative, and fulfilling. This minute holds a reward that you can carry into the future.

Today, do whatever has to be done, and do it now.

*Today's Action Plan: I will not postpone any part of my take-charge program for a thinner, healthier life. I will act now.*

*Remember, motions are the precursors of emotions. You can't control the latter directly, but only through your choice of motions—or actions.*
                                        *—Dr. George W. Crane*

The message is clear: Go through the right motions today and you'll soon begin to feel the corresponding emotions. If you smile, you'll feel happier. If you eat right, you'll feel thinner, and you'll feel in control.

You may wonder, "Why should I go around with a false grin on my face if I feel awful? Because it's more productive to work at being happy than it is to work at being grim. Positive action will create positive emotions. Abstain from overeating, and you'll feel happier and lose pounds.

Whenever you make a choice today, ask yourself, "Is this a positive action?" You'll grow more confident, effective, and successful as the pounds drop away to reveal an energized you underneath.

Motion equals emotion. Today, if your action is constructive, you will feel good about who you are.

*Today's Action Plan: I will be the manager of my emotions.*

*Make sure that what you aspire to accomplish is worth accomplishing, then throw your whole vitality into it.*
                                        *—B. C. Forbes*

The ninth action principle says, "Take weight loss in steps." That commonsense idea can get lost in the natural desire to be instantly thin. We often give ourselves deadlines for achieving a goal. But permanent weight loss results from setting one small goal, reaching it, setting the next small goal, and so on. It is a process, a journey.

Success is not measured in days, but by accomplishments. In the past you lived by the calendar and were vulnerable to imaginary failures. "After all the time I spent on this diet," you said, "I should have lost more." Such frustration puts you in danger of overeating again.

Today, set small, reachable weight-loss goals so you can experience a series of successes. You are now following your own goals.

*Today's Action Plan: I will set weight goals that I can attain, one after the other. I will put no time limits on my success.*

## July 21 — Going All the Way

*One can go a long way after one is tired.*
*—French proverb*

A successful author once said: "There are mornings when I dread facing my typewriter. I procrastinate, rearrange the pens on my desk, stare out the window. Finally, I just make a start. To my surprise, these are often my most productive days."

It's hard some mornings to face a disciplined day with healthy eating, exercise, and attention to developing more comfortable mental attitudes. But from past self-knowledge, you know you must accomplish your goals or you're going to feel far worse.

You are stronger now than ever before. When you think you can't face another day of eating right, you can. When you think you can't exercise, you can. When you believe you can't change your life, you can.

Today, remember that nothing makes you feel better

about yourself than doing what is right for your body and your life.

*Today's Action Plan: I will go farther no matter how tired I am. I will believe I can do what I must.*

**July 22**                                    **Reject Rejection**

*Unjust criticism is a disguised compliment. It often means that you have aroused jealousy and envy.*
                                        —*Dale Carnegie*

The tenth principle in your action plan says, "Reject rejection firmly and totally." We've often allowed criticism and rejection to almost destroy us. How many times have you overeaten because of a hostile sneer, a sharp word, or an unkind look?

You can cope with criticism. You can shrug it off firmly and totally, or you can do what oysters do.

Oysters handle irritation well. When an irritating grain of sand works its way inside the shell, the oyster covers it, protecting itself, while forming a beautiful pearl in the process.

When an irritant gets under your skin, make a pearl; cover it over with the triumphant, take-charge life you're living. Imagine yourself creating a glowing pearl that no criticism or rejection can ever destroy.

Today, refuse to allow any destructive criticism or rejection to get under your skin.

*Today's Action Plan: I will reject rejection. I will make a pearl out of the criticisms of today.*

*It is not true that suffering ennobles the character; happiness does that . . . suffering for the most part makes men petty and vindictive.*

                                        *—W. Somerset Maugham*

Dwelling upon your former unhappy overeating life is not wise. But it's worthwhile occasionally to remember overeating as something you certainly don't want to repeat.

Overeating drained you of everything you might have had: health, self-esteem, motivation to try for anything better.

You knew you were sick in some way, but you were too embarrassed to ask for help. You denied that you were compulsive about food and you blamed your weight on others. You felt humiliated in public most of the time.

All this suffering was the result of overeating. When you stopped overeating, the sick unhappiness left with the pounds, leaving health, self-esteem, the desire to achieve, and aliveness.

Today, realize how far you've come and become determined to go farther.

*Today's Action Plan: I will remind myself of the unhappy past, just so each today will be unforgettably good.*

*I beg you do not be unchangeable.*

                                            *—Sophocles*

Overeaters too often think they are incapable of self-improvement. Action principle eleven says, "Don't fight inevitable change." This action principle urges you to open yourself to hope, which is the catalyst in your weight-losing formula.

Perhaps in the past you saw yourself as a failure. This kind of hopeless mind-set slams the door on new information and new opportunities for change.

Change is inevitable. You can't shut it out, so use it. Try new exercises. Try new foods. Learn to love change—it gives us a chance to choose something better for our lives.

Today, see change as your hope for a thinner, healthier future. Rather than being a threat, change is an exciting new friend.

*Today's Action Plan: I will not fight inevitable change. I will open myself to everything new, hopeful, and exciting.*

## July 25                                   It's Never Ideal

*It's never ideal, and that's part of the kick, the fun of performing—improvising your way out of a hole!*
—*Eliot Fisk*

You may not be a world-renowned performer, but you share their problems. You, too, have to perform each day with circumstances that are never ideal.

Some days people don't respond to you as you wish they would. Your self-esteem is no longer based on their approval, but it would be nice if they paid you more attention. Some days you're just plain tired, cranky, and balky.

Situations are never ideal, but that's part of the challenge of a take-charge life. What would be the challenge, or the reward, if it all came easily?

You have the fun of performing on your instrument

—your body—every day. Today, see that you can perform well, no matter how trying the circumstances.

*Today's Action Plan: Ideal or not, I will make today
work for me. I will not allow any circumstance to stop
me.*

## July 26                                    Play to Win

*Success is the reward for accomplishment.*
*—Harry F. Banks*

"Play life to win," declares the twelfth principle of
your action plan. No one suggests that you step over
anyone to climb to success—simply don't defeat yourself.

Overeaters have plenty of energy, often negative
energy. We cry, "What's the use? I can't do it!" But you
can convert defeatism into victorious energy that urges,
"Keep going! Move ahead!"

Who are the people you admire? Who are the men
and women you want to be like? Whether they are successful in weight loss, in business, or elsewhere, they are
amazingly alike: Winners learn from failure, are self-
constructive critics, never blame luck or others, persist
no matter what, and experiment with change. You, too,
can play life to win.

Today, channel your energy into the winning kind of
life you admire in others.

*Today's Action Plan: I will turn negative energy into
positive energy. I will think like a winner, act like a
winner, be a winner.*

*Persistence and determination alone are omnipotent.*
*—Calvin Coolidge*

Do this one thing: make your persistence even stronger than your desire. Your most powerful positive energy is your persistence. You can't buy it; you can't borrow it; you can't inherit it—you must act on it.

You already have an achievement-prone personality. That is one of the reasons you are in such mental anguish over your weight.

If you want to be thin for life, you have to act like a winner every day of your life. Take those characteristics you admire in winners, make them yours, and act on them.

Today, believe that persistence, going one step farther, is the most important element of your personality. Nurture it and make it grow!

*Today's Action Plan: I will be persistent in all that I do. I will believe that I can do far more than I think I can.*

*It takes what it takes.*
*—Alcoholics Anonymous saying*

Some people gain ten pounds and panic while others put on a hundred pounds before the pain propels them into action. People have different levels of pain tolerance, but all overeaters can find a solution when they discover a new way to see the world and their place in it.

The negative compulsive personality is marked by passiveness, anxiety, perfectionism, supersensitivity, and sadness behind a happy facade. Compulsive overeaters buffer these feelings with excess food.

To win your new body, mind, and life, you must experience a complete psychic change. Each day you must become more action-oriented, more confident, more able to learn from mistakes and begin again, more able to reject rejection, and more emotionally honest with yourself and others.

Today, resolve to make a constructive psychic change, so that you will never have to use excess food to help you face another day.

*Today's Action Plan: I will be constructively addicted today. I can use my tendency toward compulsiveness to change my life.*

## July 29 — Recipe for Success

*Take the obvious, add a cupful of brains, a generous pinch of imagination, a bucketful of courage and daring, stir well, and bring to a boil.*
*—Bernard M. Baruch*

Sometimes the obvious is hardest to see. For overweight people, it's a set of tools—food intake charts, menu and behavior diaries, and exercise logs. Don't ignore tools that have proved helpful in the past. Incorporate them into your successful new plan for healthy eating, exercise, and take-charge attitudes.

Be ready to reuse old tools and learn new ones too. After you've lost your excess pounds, weight will no longer be an immediate problem. You'll have extra time, energy, and creative mind-power to spend on other activities.

Today, look back and use the tools that worked for you before, but be ready to learn new skills for the day when being overweight is no longer your most important problem.

*Today's Action Plan: I will use whatever tools help me.
I will think of the wonderful opportunities ahead.*

*The great pleasure in life is doing what people say you
cannot do.*
> —*Walter Bagehot*

Even the most well-meaning people can unintention-
ally sabotage our goals: "Don't you think you're getting
a little *too* thin?" Because we have changed, others feel
threatened. Therefore, assure your family and friends
that, even though you're changing your weight and
your life, they are more important to you than ever.

Watch out for the most persistent saboteur of all—
you. Don't sabotage yourself by shifting your weight
goal as you approach it, making it unattainable. Don't
sabotage your weight goal by demeaning it as you come
close, so that reaching it is no triumph.

You can't let others, or yourself, sabotage your goal of
a thin body and physical and mental fitness. Be a friend
to yourself. The payoff is a marvelously energized way
of life.

Today, reassure those who may try to sabotage your
weight-loss program because they feel uncomfortable
with your changes.

*Today's Action Plan: I won't let anyone sabotage my
weight goal, and I won't sabotage it, either.*

*The search for truth is really a lot of good fun.*
> —*Vernon Howard*

Thank yourself for caring enough to give yourself

another chance, and for your increased vitality. Thank yourself for the new confidence that got rid of old fears, and for the desire to win. Thank yourself for taking a new course, and for setting achievable weight goals. Thank yourself for the idea that you can play life to win.

Accept the responsibility to keep positive structure in your life: eat for weight loss, exercise for health, and practice attitudes of self-respect.

When you do what you know you should do, you are self-trusting, free from the fear that you will overeat. You feel a sense of peace and security.

Today, thank the one uniquely wonderful person responsible for your winning life: yourself.

*Today's Action Plan: I will remember that I am my best friend. I will not exchange the peace and security of today for any food on earth.*

AUGUST

**August 1**                    **Dream, and It Might Come True**

*Imagination is more important than knowledge.*
                                        —*Albert Einstein*

If we are what we eat, then most certainly we are what we think. Everything you imagine has an incredible power for positive or negative impact.

If you use your imagination negatively, you are poisoning your mind against yourself. When you tell yourself, "I can't do that," you're hiding fantastic capability behind negative images.

If you believe constructively, daydream affirmatively, you're priming yourself for the achievement that will be yours. Use that energy to form a positive, affirming image of yourself. Put your imagination to work for you.

Today, learn and practice positive imagination until it is yours.

*Today's Action Plan: I will imagine a new life for myself. I will take charge of my imagination and get rid of the "I can'ts."*

**August 2**                                        **Aliveness**

*Do not mistake what your life work is; it is your life.*
                                        —*Jo Coudert*

Enthusiasm boosts your sense of aliveness. The word

*enthusiasm* comes from a Greek word meaning "to be possessed by the god." Become possessed by enthusiasm—if you *act* enthusiastic, you can't help but *be* enthusiastic.

You can measure your aliveness another way. How much do you want to learn today? How many things do you want to do today? If you are eager to learn and eager to get into action, you tingle with aliveness.

Today rests firmly in your hands; today you can be as alive as you make up your mind to be. You and only you can live your life.

*Today's Action Plan: I will look back on this day and say "How alive I was!" I will let the god of enthusiasm come alive in me.*

## August 3                    The Caffeine Consequence

*The best way out is always through.*

—*Robert Frost*

Sooner or later you'll have to make a conscious health decision about caffeine. Because dieters sometimes use over-the-counter diet pills and drink diet cola, coffee, and tea that contain caffeine, they may consume higher doses of this drug than the average person. You're familiar with caffeine's side effects such as insomnia, restlessness, irritability, nervous tremors, and headaches, but there are other caffeine consequences for overeaters.

In small doses, caffeine serves as a mild stimulant. But if you overdo it, caffeine can produce mood, anxiety, and sleep disorders. That's bad news for overeaters who are trying to channel their thinking into positive mental activities.

Today, examine your caffeine intake and any negative side effects it may be causing. Then make a conscious decision to get rid of any deterrent to your winning life.

*Today's Action Plan: I will look for real energy in healthy eating and exercise. I will get rid of any substance that can keep me from my goals.*

## August 4                                   Next Time

*You become a champion by fighting one more round.*
*—James J. Corbett*

As an overweight person, you are probably a tough taskmaster with yourself. If friends have off days or make mistakes, you rush to their defense; you reassure them and try to help them. But if the errant person is you, you probably jump on yourself with both feet.

If you don't complete your plans for today, give yourself a next time. If you set a goal and miss it, give yourself a next time.

Talk back to that negative critic inside you. When it says, "You're whipped, you'll never be thin," answer right back, "That's not true!" Your negative voice expects failure. When it speaks, remember there is no such thing as total failure—not today, not in a lifetime.

Today, if you don't reach your goal, answer the bell for the next round.

*Today's Action Plan: I will talk back to my negative critic. I will give myself a next time whenever I need it.*

## August 5                              Why You Feel Bad

*Every bad feeling you have is the result of your distorted negative thinking.*
*—Dr. David D. Burns*

There's an interesting cause-and-effect aspect to bad moods. You probably believed that your depression caused negative thinking, but quite the opposite is true: Negative thinking caused your bad feelings.

Some of us have such a negative fix that we don't even realize when we are thinking negatively. When something good happens to us, we say: "That's just a fluke, a mistake. It doesn't count."

Turn off automatic negative thinking and take control of your own direction. You can take off weight if you program "I'm worth it" into your thought pattern. There's a first-class person in you.

Today, see how destructive thoughts cause your bad feelings and not vice versa. Head into the sunshine and stay there.

*Today's Action Plan: I will think that I'm a first-class person; therefore, I will be a first-class person.*

## August 6                    Puppets or Puppeteers

*Life affords no higher pleasure than that of surmounting difficulties, passing from one step of success to another, forming new wishes and seeing them gratified.*
—*Dr. Samuel Johnson*

In a puppet show, the dolls sometimes are so lifelike that you forget someone is pulling the strings. When the show ends and the puppeteer releases control, the puppets collapse without a life of their own. Similarly, your body is a puppet and your mind the puppeteer.

You are attached to your puppeteer-mind by invisible strings of thought. If your thoughts are constructive, your role will be creative; if destructive, you will fall in a heap.

Each day brings you closer to the thinner, energized body and mind you want. Each day the master puppeteer, your positive self, forms new goals and goes after them. Make today's show a celebration of your triumphant life.

Today, see how your mind guides your body. Your life is a series of thoughts acted out.

*Today's Action Plan: I will be a master puppeteer of the good life. I will pull my own strings.*

## August 7        Doubters Unmasked

*If you would have things come your way, run after them.*

*—Anonymous*

If you want success, be a doer, not a doubter. Doubters think nothing will work, so why try? They are masters of negative energy. They don't want much out of life; they don't expect much; and they become very good at negative expectations.

Although doubters appear to be aggressive, they are really very passive and fearful. Don't listen to doubters, especially the doubter in yourself.

When you were a child, you possessed great enthusiasm for trying new things. You had curiosity and faith in yourself. You were a doer, not a doubter, and you will be a doer again.

Today, see how doubting destroys enthusiasm for living. You are determined to be a doer.

*Today's Action Plan: I will not listen to doubters. I will have the self-trust and faith that I had as a child.*

## August 8        Let Go

*A great burden falls away if we let God run the universe.*

*—Robert Cummings*

Some overeaters escape the wreckage of their own lives by managing everyone else's. They don't contribute to others' welfare solely out of compassion, but find escape in good works. They have time, energy, and advice for everyone else, but their own lives are falling apart.

Are you trying to run everything—others' lives, the whole universe? Scattering all your energy on others as a cover-up for not facing yourself is a losing proposition.

What energy we use to smother the mental conflict between what we know and what we do! It's important to help others in need, but to do so you must take care of your own problems first.

Today, realize that if you dissipate all your energy to take charge of others' lives, you are not in charge of your own.

*Today's Action Plan: I will put my own house in order and leave the universe to God. I will concentrate on setting my own life straight.*

---

**August 9**                           **Act Smart**

*All the world's a stage, And all the men and women merely players.*

*—William Shakespeare*

We are all actors. In the morning we put on our costumes and get our faces ready. Then we step out into the world and perform. We smile, gesture, deliver lines. Our audience is made up of our employers, co-workers, family members, and friends.

But actors, even the finest professionals, must have a good script for a good performance. They must study and memorize their lines and deliver them with their best effort.

You know what it takes to win applause from yourself and your audience. Study the lines, memorize them, and then act them out with all your heart. You're ready for your new thin role.

Today, start acting the way you want to be. You have discovered the right role and the right lines to become a winner.

*Today's Action Plan: I will walk out on the stage of life and act like a winner. I know I will be a winner because now I have the right lines.*

**August 10**                                    **Relax and Recharge**

*When your day is largely made up of energetic, concentrated effort, provide for periods of complete relaxation when you can take it easy and recharge your batteries.*
*—Glenville Kleiser*

When we rid our days of excess food, we reduce tension, stress, and strain. But often we are in jeopardy of plunging too fast into our new life of physical and mental fitness. If you are living days of highly concentrated effort, be sure to include daily relaxation.

What helps you to relax physically and mentally? Do you like to read, or take a walk, or lie on your back in the grass? Do whatever helps you feel free from strain and at ease with your mind and body.

Each day, give yourself some time to renew your strength and energy. This will keep your enthusiasm high so you can do what you want even better. The few moments you spend unwinding will yield great benefits.

Today, rejuvenate your spirit with a rest period.

*Today's Action Plan: I will make time to relax and be at ease with myself. I will refresh myself for what I must accomplish with the rest of the day.*

*The most important thing in our lives is what we are
doing now.*

                                    *—Anonymous*

Most people believe overweight people consume a
wide variety of foods, that we are gourmets, if you will.
But in reality, most of us have a limited eating "vocabulary." We eat a small variety of the wrong things: foods
laden with fat, sugar, and salt.

You're not stuck with yesterday's food choices. The
most important thing in your life is what you're eating
today, and today you're changing your eating vocabulary to include healthier foods.

Yesterday's choices don't count; today's do, and today
you're going to ask for the right foods to energize your
new life.

Today, change your eating vocabulary to reflect the
real you that is emerging.

*Today's Action Plan: I will drop the words sugar, fat,
and salt from my eating vocabulary. I will eat for a
healthy body.*

*We are happy because we smile.*

                             *—William James*

Which comes first, the smile or happiness? According
to the law of cause and effect, we should smile after we
become happy. But we actually control our own happiness because we control our smiles.

Try this: stand in front of a mirror and smile. Keep
on doing it, even if you're depressed. You'll find you can
change your attitude by changing your action. The
more you smile, the more you feel like smiling.

You become what you do. If you smile and stand tall, you become a happier, more confident person. It's as simple as that.

Today, smile. You can't be depressed with a smile on your face. Your smile may not be real at first, but soon you won't be able to stop the happiness.

*Today's Action Plan: I will smile more. I will stand straight and tall.*

## August 13                    A Label You Can Live With

*Worry never robs yesterday of its sorrows; it only saps today of its strength.*

*—A. J. Cronin*

Size labels hurt. They start in the schoolyard: "Hey, fat stuff!" In teen years, you may have heard, "If you'd only take off weight, you could have a date for the dance." Later still, "Sorry about that promotion, but we need a different image." You're sick of being stereotyped because of your size.

Let go of those unhappy memories. Today is the day to shop for a different kind of label—a new, proud label you can wear for the rest of your life.

Find your new labels: worthy, achiever, confident, thin, healthy, winner. Now apply these labels to yourself without hesitation. You will begin to behave in these new ways.

Today, no longer worry about old labels. You have found labels that fit you now, and you wear them with pride.

*Today's Action Plan: I will not allow yesterday's labels to sap today of the strength I need. I will wear only my own labels.*

*I tried a dozen exercise programs, but I really did best
with an at-home program that I made up myself.*
                                        —*Diet club speaker*

Exercise doesn't have to be hard work. You can
achieve physical fitness with a moderate level of intensity. You don't have to jog to the office, run a marathon,
or strain on an exercise machine. You don't even have to
leave your home if you don't want to.

Try these at-home exercises: jog in place or from
room to room, dance to fast music, bounce on a small
trampoline, pedal an exercise bike, skip rope.

As with all exercise, start slowly, then increase your
speed, duration, and repetitions as you improve your
condition. Just twenty minutes each day will help you
lose weight and keep it off. You'll be stronger, your
blood pressure and heart rate will decrease, and your
disposition will be sunnier.

Think of all the energy trapped in your body. Invest
some of it in yourself today. Get moving and get thinner.

Today, try exercising for fitness and weight loss in
your own home.

*Today's Action Plan: I will do one or more of the at-
home exercises. I will get moving and keep moving.*

*My very walk should be a jig.*
                                        —*William Shakespeare*

A group of women recently participated in an experiment. All were overweight and, as the researchers put
it, resistant to diets. They were asked to do only one

thing: walk half an hour a day for one year. No pills, no lectures, no diets. They ate what they wanted.

What was the payoff after a year? An average weight loss of twenty-two pounds per person!

Walking is the easiest exercise to stick to month after month because it's something you do naturally. It's easy to fit more walking into your day—try leaving the car at home for short trips, or park a few blocks from your destination and walk.

Best of all, walk with your mate or friend. It's a wonderful way to socialize and share your thoughts while achieving a winner's fitness.

Today, begin to lose weight and improve fitness by simply walking.

*Today's Action Plan: I will walk today for at least thirty minutes. I will exercise to be a winner.*

**August 16**                    **Have You Grown?**

*The great aim of education is not knowledge but action.*

*—Herbert Spencer*

We overeaters strive to grow. The great accomplishment for us is not looking back to see how far we've come, nor looking ahead to see how far we've got to go, but growth itself. We grow as we learn. However, what we learn here or elsewhere means nothing unless we use it.

Action is the focus of our attention. It's nice to see that we're more attractive, thinner, more energetic, and successful. But we can't stop here. We must continue to do the things that got us this far. We must keep growing to win or we will zoom backward almost at the speed of sound.

Today, congratulate yourself on your wonderful

growth; you are healthier, happier, and more successful.

*Today's Action Plan: I will grow by continuing to take action.*

## August 17 A Calming Thing

*He who cannot change the very fabric of his thought will never be able to change reality.*
—Anwar al-Sadat

Anger is destructive. It may move us to seek revenge. But overeaters often take revenge on themselves by spite-eating. How many pounds do you owe to anger?

You can handle anger constructively. Anger channeled into a spirit of competition can improve your performance. This is using a negative emotion to your advantage. But if you are unable to turn a negative to a positive, calmness and serenity is a far better response to anger than eating.

To put yourself into a serene state, try repeating some calming words—a mantra, a bit of poetry, a prayer. Try to turn anger into a competitive response, or seek the calm, serene center that is in you.

Today, don't let anger force you into a fit of overeating. Extra pounds on you don't solve problems.

*Today's Action Plan: I will not eat out of spite. I will find the calm core of serenity within me.*

## August 18 Helping Others Accept Your Change

*Those who bring sunshine to the lives of others cannot keep it from themselves.*
—Sir James M. Barrie

When you begin to change before your family's eyes, it can upset the intricate family balance. You have had a particular place in this system, physically and emotionally. Changing your appearance and showing take-charge behavior can rock the family boat.

Some families get very upset. Children can feel abandoned when a permissive parent suddenly shows a healthy self-respect. Spouses can long for the return of their nonthreatening mates.

Your family needs your help, and you can give it. Let them know you really rely on their loving support. Reassure them that you're happier and that you all will be happier together now that you're not overeating. You'll help yourself and them as well.

Today, reinforce your take-charge attitudes by helping others accept them. Your relationships will change for the better.

*Today's Action Plan: I will help my family accept my change. I will no longer overeat to comfort others.*

**August 19**                                   **Friendly Persuasion**

*The trouble with most people is that they think with their hopes or fears or wishes rather than with their minds.*

*—Will Durant*

Surveys show that one-third of your support, or hindrance, when you lose weight and change attitudes comes from friends and co-workers. When you begin to change, you realize for the first time that you influence everyone around you.

It is human for others to want to be able to count on what they know. When you lose weight and change the way you view yourself in the world, even the most well-meaning friends can feel threatened. They may even say, "I liked you a lot better when you were heavier."

Reassure them that what you are doing doesn't affect your friendship with them. Tell them how important these changes are to you. It won't take long for real friends to accept and admire your efforts.

Today, help your friends accept your change. If they balk because they've lost an eating buddy, walk away.

*Today's Action Plan: I will continue my new way of viewing the world and my place in it. I will avoid those who cannot accept my new image.*

## August 20            The Perfectionist

*You will settle for nothing short of a magnificent performance in anything you do, so you frequently end up having to settle for just that—nothing.*
          *—Dr. David M. Burns*

If overeaters often are perfectionists, why don't we lose weight? As perfectionists, we usually fail to focus on a single goal. Our desire to show the world how truly worthy we are causes us to overextend ourselves, spending energy on too many diverse goals.

Perfectionists want everything at once. They find fault with others and impose impossible levels of excellence on themselves. They are unable to forgive mistakes, especially their own.

For the overweight person who feels inadequate, scared, and insecure, perfectionism is a desire to be above criticism. There is no such place, and when we seek it, we fail to take risks or make changes.

Today, see perfection as a standard, not a goal. Perfectionism obscures the real process of winning, which is action and change.

*Today's Action Plan: I will forgive others' mistakes. I will forgive my own mistakes and be patient with myself.*

*Almost all negative feelings inflict their damage only as a result of low self-esteem.*

*—Unknown*

Marilyn Monroe and Ernest Hemingway, two world-famous people, killed themselves. No one could understand why. Apparently they had everything—money, fame, talent, adoration—everything except a sense of their own self-worth.

Feelings don't always reflect reality. And the worse you feel, the more your thoughts are distorted. When you think with your feelings, everything seems out of proportion, exaggerated, and overwhelming.

You can't help feeling hurt now and then, but you can help how long you feel hurt. When you begin to express exaggerated feelings, cancel them with reality checks. You may feel hurt for the moment, but you're not going to let negative feelings get you down for long.

Feelings and reality don't always match. Today, separate the two in your mind.

*Today's Action Plan: I will keep my self-esteem high so that hurt feelings will not lead me to overeat.*

*Never let yesterday use up too much of today.*
*—Will Rogers*

Guilt nags at the conscience and creates the need to cover it up. We overeaters have a special way of hiding guilt—we bury it under piles of food.

Take charge of your guilt by asking yourself, "Am I really to blame?" Because you often see yourself as wrong and inadequate, you actually assume someone else's guilt or create guilt where none exists.

Suppose for a minute that you did something wrong and you should feel guilty. After you make apologies or restitution, there is nothing more you can do but forgive yourself. Continuing to pay and pay, usually by overeating, can't possibly improve things.

Spend today on your new life of healthy eating, exercise, and positive mental attitudes. Nothing gets rid of yesterday's guilt like living today well.

Today, realize that old guilt can't be hidden under excess food.

*Today's Action Plan: If I am to blame for any wrong, I will make amends. Then I will let go of my guilt and get on with a good life.*

## August 23                                              The Sting

*The people who get on in this world are the people who get up and look for the circumstances they want; and, if they can't find them, make them.*
                                              George Bernard Shaw

According to the laws of aerodynamics, the bumblebee, because of its heavy body and short wingspan, shouldn't be able to fly. But the bumblebee doesn't know about this law and flies anyway.

Ideal conditions don't exist for bumblebees, or for people either. We have to fly with what we've got. If conditions in your life are not ideal for eating right to lose weight, make the conditions right. Success may be knocking at your door, but you're going to have to let it in.

Don't let anything stand in your way. If, as in the case of the bumblebee, everything points to your inability to fly, fly anyway.

Today, even if conditions aren't right for you to take charge of your life, do it anyway.

*Today's Action Plan: I will make the conditions I need to eat right. I will fly.*

## August 24                    Hiding from the Truth

*It is never too late to be what you might have been.*
*—George Eliot*

We overeaters play mirror tricks; we don't look in them or we only look from the neck up and ignore our bodies. What a hopeless task, hiding from truth.

It is devastating to think of spending your life hiding from your own image. You can still be what you might have been. Don't block your own way; stand aside and let your desire to be thin overwhelm you.

Your greatest achievements are ahead of you. You do know the way; instinctively you understand what is right for your body: eat right for weight loss and health, exercise to energize your day, and practice positive can-do attitudes.

Today, quit hiding yourself from yourself and invite the truth into your life.

*Today's Action Plan: I will not be a barrier to success. I will be what I might have been.*

## August 25                    Walk On

*True enjoyment comes from activity of the mind and exercise of the body; the two are united.*
*—Alexander Humboldt*

Are your thoughts about exercise real or distorted? Do you worry about looking foolish as you stride around the neighborhood? Try adopting this attitude: I want to walk for exercise, and I'm going to do it no matter what others may think.

Exercise for pleasure and for weight loss. If you're shy about exercising in front of others, try walking before the streets are crowded.

Starting early has another advantage. Walking before breakfast seems to create *faster weight loss*. It may be that walking with an empty stomach makes the body dip into its calorie reserves. One group of women who walked thirty minutes before breakfast, in addition to an evening walk, lost 42 percent more than a group that walked only in the evening.

Today, confront distorted thinking that tells you everyone is watching what you do. You've decided to exercise when the time is right for you.

*Today's Action Plan: I will exercise without worrying about others' perceptions.*

## August 26                                    Independence

*Let fortune do her worst, whatever she makes us lose, as long as she never makes us lose our honesty and our independence.*

*—Alexander Pope*

Being truly independent means increasing your personal options. An independent, self-maintaining, self-governing person chooses to control his or her thinking, feeling, and actions.

Independence doesn't mean going it alone or isolating yourself from others. Instead, the more you think and act for yourself, the closer you can be to others because a healthy equality exists.

Each day you don't overeat is a day when you are more of an independent, self-governing person. Increasing your independence from overeating motivates you to make other wise choices, and making wise choices brings you contentment and happiness.

Today, see that to be independent is to be self-governing, which gives you the widest possible range of choices in your day.

*Today's Action Plan: I will grow toward independence by practicing self-discipline.*

**August 27**            **The One Attitude that Is You**

*. . . the best way to define a man's character would be to seek out that particular mental or moral attitude in which, when it came upon him, he felt most deeply and intensely active and alive. At such moments there is a voice inside which speaks and says, "This is the real me!"*

—*William James*

One belief that is central to your existence says, "I can live today without overeating." Confirm this belief by your action every day.

While you were overeating you asked yourself the wrong question: "Do I want to eat this?" Now you are asking the right questions: "Do I want these excess pounds?" "Do I want to feel miserable?" "Do I want this kind of future?"

These right questions are part of reality thinking. It's looking past the supposed pleasure of the next bite to the consequences of overeating *before* you eat.

Ask the right questions. Deal with reality. Now you have made yourself available for success by removing the love of excess food from your life.

Today, identify the attitude that is really you and confirm it by action.

*Today's Action Plan: I will ask myself the right questions when tempted to overeat.*

## August 28           The Overeater's Personality

*Each of us needs time for mental self-renewal.*
         *—Whitt N. Schultz*

Seven personality traits have often been identified with overeaters. How many apply to you?

1. *Low frustration tolerance*—every frustration they experience must give way to immediate satisfaction, usually food.

2. *Grandiosity*—they appear to have elevated self-regard to hide low self-esteem.

3. *Isolation*—they are insecure loners.

4. *Oversensitivity*—they take themselves too seriously and are easily hurt.

5. *Impulsivity*—they are sprinters, not marathon runners.

6. *Defiance*—"No one can tell me I can't eat chocolate!"

7. *Dependence*—they are dependent on food as well as others.

If you see yourself possessing any of these overeater traits, make positive changes. Self-confidence replaces grandiosity; caring for others replaces isolation; developing a sense of self-worth replaces oversensitivity; setting goals replaces impulsiveness; firmly rejecting rejection replaces defiance; take-charge attitudes replace dependence.

You know that you are what you do. Today, replace a negative trait with a positive one.

*Today's Action Plan: I will make positive personality changes. I will make today an emotional success.*

*Look to this day, for it is life, the very life of life.*
                                        —*Sanskrit proverb*

You're tougher than you know. Because we overeaters are sensitive to the hurts we've felt, we convince ourselves and others that we should be treated carefully. You've been hurt, but you're not fragile.

Adversity is a challenge that brought you to this day. You can make it anything you want with your positive thoughts and acts. Just as negative attracts negative, positive attracts positive. If you treat yourself as the person you want to be, you'll become that person.

Use your achieving attitudes, strengthened by your survivor's instincts. Start with your desire, then do the right physical and mental activities that will propel you to success. Your action today will turn desire into reality.

Today, find ways to handle adversity and come up fighting.

*Today's Action Plan: I will never quit. I will use every minute of this day to propel myself toward success.*

*Keep in the sunlight.*
                                        —*Benjamin Franklin*

It's tempting to think of yourself as only an overweight person, but don't let your weight rule your self-esteem. If you haven't shed the weight you wanted to in the time you've allotted, don't make yourself miserable.

When our script doesn't play the way we write it, we overeaters suffer self-blame and self-humiliation. The antidote is to look inside to find our positive selves and believe that we are far stronger than our fears.

When you're facing such feelings of failure, focus

your emotional energy on your value, and think, "I'm doing something great!"

Today, recognize that you are not defined by your weight, and your self-esteem isn't ruled by your scale.

*Today's Action Plan: I will bask in the emotional sunlight of self-worth. I will look deep inside and find strengths I didn't know I had.*

## August 31                    Give Yourself Recreation

*People who cannot find time for recreation are obliged sooner or later to find time for illness.*
*—John Wannamaker*

Recreation is essential to emotional health. It re-creates energy, quickens motivation, increases mental fitness, brings pleasure, and supplies fond memories.

Overeating, on the other hand, is not a pleasure; it doesn't leave fond memories. Can you call that uncomfortable, stuffed feeling, that disappointment in yourself, that anguish over weight gain healthy, motivating, energizing, or pleasurable?

Learn to laugh, love yourself, be comfortable in your own company. It doesn't matter what you do for recreation as long as you do it. People who can laugh, love, and enjoy themselves develop deep confidence and faith in themselves.

Today, experience the pleasurable benefits of recreation. Become a person who laughs and loves and can find joy alone or with others.

*Today's Action Plan: I will give myself pleasure through recreation—without excess food. I will seek recreation because it is essential to my health.*

**September 1**                    **Your Basic Needs and
                                    How to Meet Them**

*Without food, I will die; without food control, I won't
live.*

*—Diet group member*

To find contentment, we need more than air, food,
water, and shelter. Most essential to our happiness are
three other basic human needs: to be loved, to be productive, and to be self-valuing.

Because these needs are basic to your sense of personal worth, inner pressure compels you to fulfill them.
But when we overeat, we destroy self-worth, productiv-
ity, and our ability to love and believe we are loved. We
stunt personal growth.

When you stop overeating, you create a climate in
which growth and change can flourish—you fulfill your
basic, human needs. When you eat right, exercise, and
embrace positive mental attitudes, you feel more comfortable with yourself.

Today, see how food abuse destroys your sense of
comfort by denying you your basic human needs.

*Today's Action Plan: I will not abuse food. I will ful-
fill my basic human needs and grow more comfortable
with myself.*

*I keep the telephone of my mind open to peace, harmony, health, love and abundance. Then, whenever doubt, anxiety, or fear try to call me, they keep getting a busy signal.*

—*Edith Armstrong*

When you're in conflict with basic needs—sustenance, safety, love, self-esteem, and creativity—anxiety results.

Overeating is an attempt to escape from anxiety, but it has only a momentary anesthetic effect. You have to eat more to control the pain of conflict, isolating yourself further from reality.

When your needs conflict, try deliberate relaxation instead of eating. Sit in a quiet room. Tense all your muscles at once: clench your fists, squeeze your eyes, clamp your teeth. Now take a deep breath, hold it for a five count, then exhale and relax your muscles for several minutes. This total relaxation is guaranteed to create a more pleasant memory than a food binge.

Today, practice real physical relaxation instead of overeating. You will have done exactly what is right for you.

*Today's Action Plan: I will not turn to food as a drug for anxiety relief. Instead I will practice relaxation.*

*The smallest action is better than the largest plan.*
—*John Graves*

Be assertive with food. We may try to laugh about succumbing to temptation ("The devil made me do it!"), but when food controls us, it's no joke.

It's time for you to be the food boss. When a high-calorie dessert calls to you from the refrigerator, quietly and firmly tell it no. We overeaters have given food power that we must take back.

Be assertive when you eat out. Once you have finished eating what is right for you, don't eat more. Politely but firmly decline to finish the dish.

Success is a habit, in this case, the habit of saying no. Don't let food or other people control your life.

Today, discover how being in control of the food you eat gives you a wonderful sense of take-charge strength.

*Today's Action Plan: I will firmly refuse any food that is not on my healthy eating plan. I will be the boss.*

**September 4**            **Take Charge of Fat in Your Food**

*The moment a question comes to your mind, see yourself mentally taking hold of it and disposing of it. Thus you learn to become the decider and not the vacillator.*
                                                    —*H. Van Anderson*

Each day you are making decisions in your life. You have truly become the driver and not just the passenger. You are creating your own winning future.

Today, decide how much fat you allow into your body. Increasing scientific evidence links fat, especially saturated fat, in food with heart disease and cancer, and some research shows it is more of a problem than sugar for overweight people.

The payoff in reducing your consumption of fat is accelerated weight loss, better health, and probably longer life.

Today, take control and make important fat-reducing decisions about your health and body.

*Today's Action Plan: I will limit my fat consumption.
I will decide that I'm in charge of my body and my life.*

## September 5 Cope-ability

*Rule No. 1 is, don't sweat the small stuff.
Rule No. 2 is, it's all small stuff.*
                                        *—Robert Eliot*

Anxiety is a fancy word for emotional pain—pain that can be very real. You can't avoid painful experiences; everyday life is full of them, especially if you're overweight. But overeating hasn't been a good barricade to emotional pain in the past—it just created its own pain.

Overeating works like iodine on a cut—it makes the hurt feel worse. Situations and people will sometimes upset you, and using food as a buffer won't help. Concentrate instead on things that will turn opportunities into reality.

Today, turn anxious moments into assets, failures into successes, defeats into victories. Any day you live without the emotional buffer of excess food, you are a winner.

*Today's Action Plan: I will remember that most of the problems that prompt me to eat are small stuff.*

## September 6 Negative I-grams

*Obstacles are those frightful things you see when you take your eyes off the goal.*
                                        *—Hannah More*

Are you so enthusiastic about your lifestyle that you won't settle for anything less? If you aren't, check your "I-grams"—the "I" instructions that form your self-image. When you telegraph negative messages to yourself, such as "I'm no good" or "I'm a fat slob," you make those messages your goal.

Don't make life decisions based on negative thinking. That's punishing yourself. Instead, be aware of how often you sabotage yourself with "I can't" thoughts.

It's against the law to mislabel a product, so package yourself right. Attach a cheerful, positive label on yourself. By sending positive "I-grams" to your self-image, you are merely obeying truth-in-packaging laws. Start right now to think, "I have what it takes to succeed."

Today, base life decisions on positive "I-grams."

*Today's Action Plan: I will give myself positive labels. I will keep my eye on my goal, a life without excess food.*

## September 7        The Convincing Self-Critic

*There are some people who are very resourceful at being remorseful.*

*—Ogden Nash*

"I am worthwhile." Are you convinced of that truth? Too often we overeaters are so angry with ourselves that we convince others of our lack of worth. With vivid language we persuade others—and ourselves—that we are rotten people. We fight any tiny sense that we have value.

Self-haters can't avoid occasional positive experiences, but when something wonderful happens, they disqualify it. It doesn't count because they don't deserve it. Their negative thinking is ingrained, so they hang on to it with all their strength.

Stop being a convincing self-critic. Refuse to persecute yourself. If you make a mistake today, think, "I'm only human, and the whole of me is not ruined." Give yourself a little peace.

Today, confront your convincing self-critic with a demand to stop this self-abuse. You deserve kindness—from yourself.

*Today's Action Plan: I will not disqualify positive experiences. I deserve the chance to succeed today.*

## September 8       How to Fight Your Inner Critic

*Expect victory and you make victory.*
                                    *—Preston Bradley*

Overeaters who make mistakes don't know when to stop blaming themselves. Their busy inner critics begin to drum out their negative messages: "You've failed again! You deserve to be fat!" This can lead to more overeating.

If you must criticize yourself, try this when you've made a mistake: Set a definite time (about five minutes) to be angry about it. Stand in front of a mirror and shout all the things your nasty inner critic has been thinking. Moan, cry, hit the walls. When the time is up, stop. The incident is ended.

You'll find that long before the end of your five-minute purge, you'll be tired of it. You don't really believe the rotten things your inner critic was saying. You're in charge of everything, even your own self-put-downs.

Today, banish your self-critic with your own scream therapy. You've sent an eviction notice to that critical drummer!

*Today's Action Plan: I will defeat my inner critic. I will take any step to gain victory over overeating.*

*[Happiness is the] agreement of a person's inner life with the reality of his outer experience.*

—*William James*

Happiness is achieved by expressing your inner values through your actions—by creating harmony between what you want (to stop overeating) and what you do (healthy eating, exercise, and attitude).

Some people have a special talent for achieving happiness. They work constantly for what they want and accept nothing less. They enjoy the excitement of challenge. They are confident in their values, and believe their lives have meaning and direction. They are self-directed, without conflict, and at peace.

You, too, are good at happiness. When you get rid of the need for excess food, you will enjoy life regardless of setbacks. You'll get more out of everything you do.

Today, put your ideals and actions in agreement by healthy eating. It is a beginning that makes future happiness possible.

*Today's Action Plan: I will develop my talent for happiness. I will get the most out of today by controlling my desire for excess food.*

*Although words exist for the most part for the transmission of ideas, there are some which produce violent disturbance in our feelings.*

—*Albert Einstein*

More than once you've heard a person say, "She doesn't mind being fat. Why, she laughs and makes jokes about it herself." But that's not the way it feels; we laugh to cover up the hurt.

It hurts to feel like an outsider, so we laugh to show it doesn't. It hurts to be excluded from the party, so we pretend we're too busy to go anyway. We may rationalize, joke, or laugh about being overweight, but that's not the way we really feel.

Today hurtful words cannot harm you. Happiness is a natural state of mind when you follow your three-part plan: healthy eating, energizing your body with exercise, and concentrating on your action plan.

Today, don't laugh to cover hurt. Instead love the real laughter that your new life is making possible.

*Today's Action Plan: I will not be disturbed by others' words. I will make happiness my natural state of mind.*

### September 11

**Help Yourself to a Bigger Portion of Life**

*Life is either daring adventure or nothing.*
　　　　　　　　　　　　*—Helen Keller*

Self-image is built from the accumulated impressions of your life, which can be changed by gathering new impressions. It is important to have the best self-image we can create because our self-image directs the way we act.

People who successfully re-create their self-image have positive attitudes, are receptive to life changes, and feel personally responsible for their own health. They can also re-create themselves physically because they are in tune with their bodies, focusing their attention on the physical changes they want to make.

Winners can create a positive self-image. You are

eating for health and happiness, piling up positive impressions for your new self-image, like a winner.

Today, gather new, positive, responsible, successful impressions.

*Today's Action Plan: I will re-create myself with a positive self-image. I will gather winning impressions.*

## September 12          Toward Personal Growth

*Underneath my mirror there's a little sign that says, "This person is not to be taken too seriously."*
            *—Dr. Lawrence Mintz*

As we've seen, being overweight in a thin-is-in culture is no laughing matter. But it doesn't do any harm if, every now and then, you take yourself and your problem just a little less seriously.

Being able to see humor in a situation is quite different from making yourself the butt of "fat jokes." If you can laugh at small obstacles, you'll find you can rebound faster and feel less frustration. Laughter is great for taking the steam out of anger, allowing your self-worth to rise.

Work on your weight problem, but see the humor around you at the same time. With a sense of humor, you'll look at your problems differently and not get so beaten down.

Today, relax and laugh a little. You will put more light moments into your day.

*Today's Action Plan: I will see the humor in life's situations. I will not take myself so seriously.*

*To the extent that a person fails to attain self-esteem, the consequence is a feeling of anxiety, insecurity, self-doubt, the sense of being unfit for reality, inadequate to existence.*

—*Nathaniel Branden*

In data processing, there's a well-known warning against careless programming: Garbage in, garbage out. What's true of a computer is true of your mind.

The lowest form of mental garbage is "Whatever I am, is wrong." With that input, you either become a doormat, begging people to step on you, or become so aggressive and unacceptable that your behavior makes you an outcast. Either way, you are apt to overeat.

Adopt a new program: "Whatever I am, is right." With your new program loaded into your memory bank, you have a solid belief in your own worth. Anxiety is replaced with confidence, and you are prepared to play life to win. Positive in, positive out.

Today, get rid of mind-garbage by reprogramming your mental computer with positive messages.

*Today's Action Plan: I will think, "Whatever I am, is right." I will put into my mind what I want to get out.*

*Half of today is better than all tomorrow.*

—*Jean de La Fontaine*

Sometimes overeaters think it's impossible to commit themselves in the morning to a full day of healthy eating. If you feel you can't make a full commitment today, don't wait until tomorrow to take action. Promise yourself you'll eat right for half a day.

Now that you've committed yourself to a half-day, you've given yourself extra time, the time you used to spend eating. Use the time to think and to create new ways to live.

Every day, even every half-day, your powerful thoughts create a winning aura around you. Don't dwell on your anxiety or depressing conditions. Not once.

You have the power to think, to create, to plan. Use it to tell yourself the truth: what you want is possible. Train yourself to think of possibilities, and when your half-day is over, you won't want to stop.

Today, give yourself at least a half-day. Half of today is more important than all of tomorrow.

*Today's Action Plan: I will use my time to create a mental environment that will help me stay free of overeating.*

**September 15**      **Do You Have Too Many Choices?**

*There are no circumstances, however unfortunate, that clever people do not extract some advantage from.*
*—François, Duc de La Rochefoucauld*

If problems are opportunities, there are a lot of opportunities around—maybe too many for overeaters choosing weight-losing methods. We have to decide between diet clubs, self-help therapy groups, spas, salons, hypnotism, clinics, books, TV diet gurus, doctors, powders, pills, shots—we are overwhelmed by alternatives.

Here's a formula to help you decide. Ask yourself:

- What do I want?
- What must I do to get it?
- Where do I go?
- When should I start?

You'll eliminate all but a few possibilities. Then give these, one at a time, a chance to work for you. But don't let indecision continue for long—it inevitably leads to overeating.

Today you are focused, functioning at a winning level. Your mind is aware, clear, and set on a goal. That makes decisions possible.

Today, take action to help you make a choice. When you have a problem, you will find a way to work it out.

*Today's Action Plan: I will make decisions as quickly and intelligently as possible. I will focus on winning my goal of mastery over food.*

## September 16                                    Winning Dreams

*Dream lofty dreams, and as you dream, so shall you become. Your vision is the promise of what you shall at last unveil.*

*—John Ruskin*

It happened like this. You picked up this book. You began to read a page, anywhere. You read it again and made a decision to start each day with a reading, giving two minutes of your time to yourself.

Before you realized it, you were hooked. You found your view of yourself and your life changing. You plunged into a new lifestyle of healthy eating, exercise, and mental fitness.

You are losing weight, you feel attractive and healthy, and your self-esteem is high. This success has expanded into other phases of your life: You win the game, land the job, become more loving. You, not food, play the leading role.

Is it right to dream such dreams? You bet it is! Now go beyond dreams. Blend them with action.

Today, dream wonderful dreams. You are ready to move beyond dreams to winning success and a new body.

*Today's Action Plan: I will dream of what I want to be. I will make these dreams reality with my action program.*

### September 17                                     Take Responsibility

*Every person is responsible for all the good within the scope of his or her abilities.*

*—Gail Hamilton*

Who are "they" that we blame? Who are the ones responsible for our bad feelings, intense anxiety, and even depression? Overeaters who avoid self-responsibility only magnify their problems. They approach life as if all events were entirely beyond their control. They feel manipulated at the hands of "they."

Take responsibility for your feelings, thoughts, and actions. If you know you need a change in your life, take responsibility for making that change. This makes more sense than living in fear of "they."

Take charge of your emotional life and build emotional strength. Know your worth. Accomplish your goals. Stand your ground. Initiate action.

Today, see that making "them" responsible for your feelings is self-destructive. Take charge of today's feelings so there will be no need to overeat.

*Today's Action Plan: I will control what happens inside me. I will express my feelings responsibly so that I will not overeat.*

*We readily welcome to our group of friends that one who talks with the voice of experience and common sense. . . . He is going to point out the pitfalls and mistakes that experience has taught him to avoid.*
—*George Matthew Adams*

Do you think being strong means going it alone? Absolutely not! In times of high stress, when you are in danger of overeating, talk to someone who is important to you. Don't turn to food; turn to a real friend, a relative, a minister, or your support group.

Overeaters cannot be islands. We must be willing to seek and accept help when we need it. Often, we receive feedback from another that helps us work out a solution. More often, we hear ourselves working out our own solutions. And we feel cared about.

Ask for all the help you need. Then take it and make necessary changes in your life. Isn't this better than being alone?

Today, don't be an island. It is so much better to turn to a helpful friend than to your food enemy.

*Today's Action Plan: I will discuss stressful events with someone important to me. I will not eat from stress.*

*The trick is not how much pain you feel. Life is full of excuses to feel pain, excuses not to live.*
—*Erica Jong*

Overeaters feel pain—the pain of living in a world that sometimes despises us, discriminates against us, and laughs at us. We have plenty of opportunities to feel righteous self-pity, but self-pity is really just an admission that we feel inadequate, helpless, and lonely.

Self-pity is a phantom pain, like the pain an amputee feels in a limb that is no longer there, a remembered pain that stops us from facing today. It becomes an excuse not to try.

Learn from the past and let it go. Drop old pain like a bad habit by understanding how destructive it is. Understanding, not awareness, is the starting point. Understanding puts you in charge of your pain, so you can choose to let it go.

Today, see that self-pity is really self-induced helplessness. Remembered pain can be an excuse not to live today to its fullest. Get rid of all self-pity.

*Today's Action Plan: I will not be diverted by yesterday's pain. I will take charge of any desire to feel sorry for myself.*

## September 20            Heart and Soul

*Strong convictions precede great actions.*
*—J. F. Clarke*

Victory in sports is achieved through the athletes' natural talent and good luck. But winning takes more than raw talent and the random bounce of a ball. Winning requires heart-and-soul commitment.

Heart-and-soul commitment is a strength and fiber of spirit. It is something inside you that makes you dig down to discover your true self and act on it.

In your daily struggle for a thinner, healthier life, you have barely touched your innate ability. Do you want to become a champion? Of course you do, with all your heart and soul!

World titles are won by fighters like you who prepare both mentally and physically to win, who dig down deep for that something extra when they need it. Believe there's a champion in you.

Today, decide to win the gold medal of life. You are ready to dig deep for that champion spirit to free yourself from overeating.

*Today's Action Plan: I will work with all my heart and soul to uncover the superstar within me.*

**September 21**  **You Are Only Responsible for Your Own Feelings**

*Mama may have, Papa may have, but God bless the child who's got his own.*

—*Billie Holiday*

Beware people who try to manipulate you with criticism. If what they say is constructive, you can respect and learn from it. But if the criticism is merely an attempt to make you conform to others' ideas, reject it.

Our rejection of their ideas might make them say, "I always give you my best, and you don't appreciate it." But don't accept responsibility for anyone else's feelings *if* you haven't done anything wrong.

Some of the negative feedback you get from others may be a disguised request for you to become what they want you to be. By gently reminding them that they are in charge of their feelings, you put the responsibility where it belongs.

You need not take charge of any feelings but your own. Be considerate of others, but maintain your own healthful self-responsibility and integrity first.

Today, firmly reject manipulative attempts to make you change. You are in charge of your own feelings.

*Today's Action Plan: I will reject attempts to make me responsible for feelings other than my own.*

*He who asks of life nothing but the improvement of his own nature is less liable than anyone else to miss and waste life.*

—*Henri-Frédéric Amiel*

You are a fabulous storehouse of valuable resources. Even if your life is beset with problems and you're at the end of your rope, you can still hang on and win. Why? Because your store of courage won't let you fall.

You can solve more problems and hang on longer because you know you can. If you believe you can achieve, you're halfway to success. Now put your confidence in action, and win.

Half a life is not for you. Move out front and earn everything you think is wonderful. Begin by getting food out of your way with healthy eating, getting your body energized and moving with your choice of exercise, and using your action plan to change the way you feel about yourself.

Today, recognize that you have the resource of courage. You will succeed because you believe you can.

*Today's Action Plan: I will plan how I want to act. I will act the way I plan.*

*It is impossible to predict what is not possible.*

—*Anonymous*

Your belief system is the result of your actions being directed by your feelings, thoughts, and attitudes. If you want something you don't have—a healthy body, for example—you must change the way you feel, think, and act.

You have the potential to become what your belief system dictates. Your positive inner force, powered by desires, pushes you toward health and confident attitudes.

Predict health and thinness, and shut out all contrary feelings and attitudes. Each day your positive, winning belief system stimulates you to grow toward your desire of a thin, energized body and a confident self-respect. Your new belief system will take you where you want to go.

Today, see how your feelings, thoughts, and attitudes formed your belief system. Adjust it, if necessary, to get the winning life.

*Today's Action Plan: I will adjust my belief system to help me become what I want to be. I will predict health and thinness.*

## September 24 **The Halo Effect**

*The anticipation of failure is a self-fulfilling prophecy.*
—*Anonymous*

Determining one's whole personality from a single characteristic results in what some psychologists call a "halo effect." For example, if you fared badly on a diet once, you might expect all diets to go badly. Anticipation of failure can be a self-fulfilling prophecy for overeaters.

The chain can be broken. If you have a negative experience, learn from it. Learning is a form of success that you can immediately reinforce.

Keep a record of the lessons you learn from negative experiences. If you fall, get up, learn the lesson, and go on to do it better the next time. You break negative chains this way.

The halo effect projects a chain reaction of failure into the future, making it come true. Today, break the chain.

*Today's Action Plan: I will not let one failure dictate my future. I will break the chain of failure by learning what went wrong.*

## September 25                    Which Road to Follow

*[The Cheshire Cat says] ". . . it doesn't matter which way you go."*
*". . . so long as I get somewhere," Alice adds.*
                                        *—Lewis Carroll*

If you don't care where you're going, any road will take you there. If you have no goal, you don't know where you're going or which road to follow.

Set a specific goal. "I want to lose weight" is not specific. "I want to lose thirty-seven pounds" is specific.

Set a positive goal. "I don't want to be fat and ugly" is not positive. "I want to lose weight so that I will be happy, healthy, and more attractive" is positive.

You do care where you're going. You have a choice between something and nothing. You know your goal. Now take the steps to self-respect and success.

Today, set specific, positive weight and living goals. Today, dig deeper and reach higher than you thought you could.

*Today's Action Plan: I will care where I'm going. I will have a goal and a way to reach it.*

## September 26                         Achieving Goals

*Laboring toward distant aims sets the mind in a higher key and puts us at our best.*
                                        *—C. H. Parkhurst*

The primary objective of this book is to help you set and achieve your life goals. And you have three: you want to control your weight, you want to re-energize your body, and you want to view life as winners do.

There are criteria for achieving these goals:
1. Set a specific, positive goal.
2. Provide effective motivation with interim goals.
3. Develop continuous effort; regularity is the key.
4. Overcome setbacks by learning from problems.
5. Recognize and celebrate small successes.

Today, set a goal and develop a plan for achieving it. You're not standing in line with your hand out. You're in charge.

*Today's Action Plan: I will set goals for myself. I will not waste my life by postponing action.*

## September 27                    Have You Got a Hunch?

*A hunch is creativity trying to tell you something.*
                                        —*Anonymous*

You've broken through the debilitating cycle of over-eating-starving-overeating through understanding and action. You are developing a strong sense of yourself. You have a hunch that something good is happening to you.

Your life is now built around a central idea—a solid understanding of your self-worth. Today, playing life to win, you are alive, joyous, and vital.

Once you looked for happiness in food, when happiness was really within you all the time. Look within yourself. You have all that you need to be a winner.

It's exciting to take charge of your life, to find you have a will of your own. Doing what needs to be done promptly is a basic part of rational living, and your life makes sense now.

Today, you have a hunch that your life is going to be wonderful, and you're right.

*Today's Action Plan: I will pay attention to my positive hunches. I will build my life on a solid understanding of my unique worth.*

## September 28                                     Just Your Luck!

*I think luck is the sense to recognize an opportunity and the ability to take advantage of it.*
—Samuel Goldwyn

"Just my luck!" you say when something goes awry. This attitude is a subtle form of self-sabotage.

Look again at the words: "Just my luck!" You are equating your luck with your self-worth, as though your luck would be better if *you* were better. With that attitude you'll see every evidence of bad luck as proof of your own unworthiness.

Luck has nothing to do with your weight. Luck is an opportunity you either take advantage of or don't. You are now holding a lucky opportunity in your hand. Will you take advantage of what you read here and apply it to your weight and living problems?

Today, make your own luck. Thinking you are singled out for bad luck is a negative game to play with your self-worth.

*Today's Action Plan: I will see opportunities as luck. I will take advantage of my lucky day.*

## September 29          Use Your Momentum for Change

*There are no permanent changes because change itself is permanent.*
—Ralph L. Woods

Most diet experts warn against trying to change other habits while you're losing weight. This may be good advice when you are just beginning weight control or if a diet is merely added to your present life, but other changes *are* possible.

You've already changed from sedentary habits to physical exercise and changed your low self-esteem to high regard.

You can use the momentum you have gained from your three-part living plan to tackle other changes you want to make, such as quit smoking, reduce alcohol consumption, change jobs, go back to school.

Once you're truly on the road to achieving a thinner, healthier body, you can continue to make good changes. And you're ready for that.

Today use the momentum and strength and confidence of your take-charge program to make other good changes in your life.

*Today's Action Plan: I will tackle other changes after I have overeating under control. I see change as a challenge.*


## September 30                           Back to Basics

*If we search for the fundamentals which actually motivate us, we will find . . . it is to some of them that we owe that big urge which pushes us onward.*
                                        *—Edward S. Jordan*

The best educators return to school for refresher courses. The great professional athletes still take coaching lessons on fundamental moves and strategy. The most talented concert pianists continue to practice their keyboard exercises.

All these people, tops in their fields, have something

in common. They realize that one must maintain the basics, the solid foundation of fundamentals on which success was built.

Recovering overeaters, too, must maintain a solid foundation of fundamentals. You know what they are: your healthy eating food plan, regular exercise, and a positive attitude. These are the basics you need to be a winner.

Today, go back to the basics of the action principles for a refresher course. As for all champions, fundamentals help you keep winning.

*Today's Action Plan: I will always act according to the fundamentals on which my new life is built.*

**October 1**                      **Diet Groups Are Not for All**

*I felt smothered by people who wanted too much of me, and who, because I had lost weight, thought I owed them everything.*

                         *—Diet group member*

Diet groups help a great many people lose weight, but they're not for everyone. Membership in any group means loss of some individuality, some freedom to think, feel, and act for ourselves. If the advantages—a supportive environment, self-understanding, education—are greater than the disadvantages, you'll be content. If not, you'll need to look further.

Visit a variety of weight-losing groups. Do you get support? Is the group too expensive? Do you see success? Does the group withdraw friendship from those who slip off the prescribed diet? Does the group attack or encourage? Does it raise successful members up and later knock them down?

Even the best group may not be for you. Or you may want to attend meetings occasionally to boost your spirits. Remember, you're in charge.

Today, use these questions to evaluate weight-loss groups, remembering that you can join a group and go regularly, occasionally, or not at all. The choice is yours.

*Today's Action Plan: I will evaluate groups carefully, making choices that decrease frustration and increase contentment.*

## October 2                 The Big Difference

*Many people go from infancy to senility without ever achieving maturity.*

*—Anonymous*

The big difference between immaturity and maturity, between dependence and independence, between a loser and a winner is self-understanding. We often call it "self-awareness," using the two terms interchangeably. Yet the terms are as different as day and night.

Self-awareness is a game we play; it shows everybody how much we know about ourselves. But it's a loser's game unless it progresses to self-understanding. Self-awareness merely says, "I know why I hurt!" Self-understanding bravely says, "This is my mess and I must clean it up myself."

Maturity is independence. When we cling to our disappointments without taking responsibility for changing them, we spend life in a helpless dither.

Today, see the difference between self-awareness and self-understanding. It's not enough just to be aware of your feelings—you must also do something about them.

*Today's Action Plan: I will not say "I hurt" without finding a way to stop hurting. I will take charge of my awareness.*

## October 3                 "No Excuse, Sir."

*The difficult we do immediately—the impossible takes a little longer.*

*—Slogan of the U.S. Army Corps of Engineers*

Anyone who has served in the military knows that alibis for failure to perform are frowned on by superior officers. The only acceptable explanation is, "No excuse, sir." Even if you have a good excuse, it's considered inappropriate to offer it. It takes a lot of self-confidence not to offer an excuse if you have one.

Self-confidence is another name for security. Practice it. Stop making excuses for possible failure in your program of healthy eating, exercise, and action. Instead, find reasons why you will succeed.

Don't get stuck in the trap of past pain. What overeating did to you isn't as important as what you do about your overeating.

Today, take total responsibility for your actions. It's the most confident thing you can do.

*Today's Action Plan: I will make no excuses. I will not overeat today, doing today what was impossible yesterday.*

## October 4                    Positive Rewards

*Learn to repeat endlessly to yourself: "It all depends on me."*

*—André Gide*

Success is setting and attaining goals. How can you ensure that you will repeat the positive behavior that brings you to your goal of physical and mental fitness? Rewarding yourself can do wonders.

We tend to repeat behavior that brings positive feedback—especially *immediate* positive feedback. Food can do that: our senses of smell, sight, and touch are immediately engaged.

What you need is immediate reinforcements for your new way of healthful eating. Make a list of positive

reinforcers: nonfood items you really enjoy, like a telephone chat with a friend or relative, reading a good
book, or listening to favorite music.

Keep records of positive eating behavior as a reinforcement. When you reach a certain goal, give yourself
an extra-special reward—new clothes, theater tickets, or
a trip.

Today, reinforce success immediately so you will continue to do what will lead to the biggest reward, your
new body and life.

*Today's Action Plan: I will give my healthy eating plan
immediate positive reinforcement. I will celebrate my
successes.*

## October 5                          Unfinished Business

*To be what we are, and to become what we are capa-
ble of becoming, is the only end of life.*
—*Robert Louis Stevenson*

When you overate, you were continually off balance.
It's as if one hand (your desire to stop) pushed against
the other (your compulsion to overeat). What is the
unfinished business of your life? What are the things
you most want to do? When you control your eating,
you are better able to control other events in your life.

You know the joy of having your life in balance, having your goals agree with what your mind tells you to
do. You have mastered the tug and pull between playing it safe and driving for success. You know the difference between the false and temporary fullness after
overeating and the real fulfillment of healthy eating.

With overeating out of the way, you can begin to
tackle the unfinished business in your life.

Today, distinguish between the stressful imbalance of

the overeater's life and the security of your healthy eating, exercise, and action attitudes.

*Today's Action Plan: I will get on with any unfinished business in my life. I will be master of what I eat.*

## October 6           Happiness Re-examined

*Happiness is the only sanction of life; where happiness fails, existence remains a mad, lamentable experiment.*
*—George Santayana*

Life has no meaning without happiness or at least some hope of attaining it. For overeaters, there can be little happiness when eating is out of control. In the past, we lived with dissatisfaction, instability, criticism, boredom, helplessness, and underutilization of our abilities. When we overate, happiness faded.

But when we choose healthy eating, exercise, and positive attitudes, the road ahead becomes smooth. A happy life becomes possible. Should we reach even half our happiness potential, we'll do better than most people.

You are capable of compulsion—so far, misdirected toward food. Paradoxically, the very compulsion that got you into trouble can make you a winner, if you turn it into a drive toward achievement.

Today, find where your true happiness lies and decide to give it your all.

*Today's Action Plan: I will never return to the hell of overeating. I will drive forward to happiness.*

*It was a real catch-22 situation. I was unhappy with*
*my diet group, but I was afraid if I didn't keep going*
*I'd regain all my weight.*
                              *—Ex-diet group member*

Many overeaters find success in self-help diet groups.
But if you become unhappy with a group for any reason, you have a perfect right to leave.

When you join a group tell yourself you will stay or
leave as you choose. Later, if you decide to withdraw, do
so without guilt or fear. To ease the strain of leaving,

1. Choose a time when you're having success in your
life, other than weight loss.

2. Announce your plan to leave ahead of time so you
can say good-bye. You don't have to sneak out.

3. Use a positive vocabulary. Rather than "dropping
out" from failure, you are "graduating" after success.

4. Believe that you have the right to continue
weight-loss independently and the right to come back
to the group later, if you choose.

Today, know that you are in charge of your life. Make
choices, and accept the responsibility.

*Today's Action Plan: I will never stay in a diet group*
*out of fear or guilt.*

*Stature comes not with height but with depth.*
                              *—Benjamin Lichtenberg*

You are a person of value. The inner you is not negative, and you're no quitter. The real you does not lack
for brains or courage.

Don't be discouraged today or any day, even if you
fall short of your capabilities. You are human. When

you are less than you know you can be, less than you want to be, be gentle with yourself. Then get to work again.

You needn't wait until your body is slender to accept your goodness. You needn't put off enjoying a new life of healthful eating, exercise, and attitudes until you are more deserving; you deserve it now.

Today, accept the fact that you are a valuable person, but human. If you falter, be sympathetic with yourself and get right back into action.

*Today's Action Plan: I will believe in my inner good. I will look for good in myself and work on the rest.*

## October 9                    Re-create Your Body

*I believe the potential for [physical] transformation is available to every human being.*
                              —*Dr. Suki Rappaport*

You are always re-creating and changing your body. You are physically different than you were five years or even one year ago.

You can channel this physical change in the direction you'd like it to go. Cooperate with your body—it wants and needs health. It is transformed with healthy eating, physical exercise, and your glowing new attitudes.

Overeating is life-threatening—it can keep you from living fully, even from feeling completely alive.

Visualize the body you want to begin creating today. Use this image to reinforce your three-part living plan, then follow this image with action. You have the power to transform your body.

Today, see that you have the power to literally grow a new body day by day.

*Today's Action Plan: I will eat, exercise, and act to re-create the body I want.*

*If you have the will to win, you have achieved half your success; if you don't, you have achieved half your failure.*

—*David V. A. Ambrose*

Too often, many of us overweight people commit a little mental suicide. We throw up our hands and say, "I just can't go on."

Surveys show that overweight people are generally less happy with themselves than thinner people. They're unhappy about their weight, but mostly about their lack of control.

We humans have little control over circumstances outside ourselves. Weather, war, economic depression—all are beyond our individual sway. But if we feel we have no influence over ourselves, we feel completely helpless and powerless.

You will be unhappy to the extent that you feel out of control. Take charge of what you eat today. Without eating control, nothing can follow. With eating control, everything falls into place.

Today, face the reason for your unhappiness. Every day that you act on your healthy eating plan will lead you to the happy life.

*Today's Action Plan: I will not kill my chance for happiness by overeating. I know that good will follow from self-control.*

*Go confidently in the direction of your dreams.*
                              *—Henry David Thoreau*

Change needs direction—your direction. You know what you want, and you have the power to get it. As always, the paramount action for you is to get over-eating out of the way so you can find what your life is meant to be.

Begin by reviewing your chosen lifestyle and the eating, exercising, and attitude changes you have made. Ask yourself:

1. "What is my problem?" (Assess your eating problem.)

2. "How does it make me feel or act?" (Assess food's negative power.)

3. "What can I do about it?" (Make your decision for today.)

4. "Will I do it?" (Make your commitment for today.)

5. "How will I achieve it?" (Evaluate and improve your plan.)

Because of your choices, you are no longer just an eating machine; you are more truly yourself.

Today, choose to be in charge of your life's direction.

*Today's Action Plan: I will set my own course. I will live my life as I imagined I would.*

*Unless a capacity for thinking be accompanied by a capacity for action, a superior mind exists in torture.*
                              *—Benedetto Croce*

Are you, despite your best efforts, sometimes haunted by thoughts of certain foods? When you are tired, hungry, and frustrated the old ways of dealing with these feelings can sneak back into your mind.

Visualize yourself acting on a food obsession. See your hand reaching for the food. Shout, "Stop!" and replace the scene with the image of you, slender, running on a country road on a crisp autumn morning.

Repeat this technique until you can shift from a desire for certain foods to an image of the ideal you. With practice, you'll be able to change thoughts at will.

As a problem-solver, you must learn to reprogram your mind for a winning lifestyle. Food fantasies are destructive. What you do is reality; and reality, not fantasy, is your friend.

Today, replace a negative thought with the image of your real self.

*Today's Action Plan: I will practice stopping negative thoughts. I will take charge of my food obsession.*

## October 13      Cold-Weather Exercise Addicts

*After eight to ten weeks you'll find yourself looking forward to your exercise, longing for it as an accustomed pleasure.*
*—Dr. Kenneth H. Cooper*

By now you may be devoted to daily exercise and feel deprived when bad weather keeps you from the outdoors. Don't despair! Switch to indoor exercises that will maintain weight loss and keep you feeling alive.

Try stationary running on a thick carpet. Use up-tempo music if you need help maintaining a steady rhythm.

Try skipping rope. It adds tone to muscles in your arms, shoulders, and chest—not a bad payoff for as little as fifteen minutes a day.

Three-step climbing is another easy, first-rate indoor exercise. Up and down three steps for five minutes can give you aerobic benefits.

Combine and vary these indoor exercises to maintain the wonderful sense of physical self you've developed through your three-part lifestyle.

Today, find a way to continue your physical program, no matter what the weather is like. You no longer look for reasons to quit, but ways to continue.

*Today's Action Plan: I will plan indoor exercise for inclement weather and will have fun doing them.*

## October 14 — Overeating Is Boring

*I never went anywhere, never did anything new. I just wanted everybody to get out of my way, so I could eat, eat, eat!*

*—Diet group member*

Too little has been written in weight-loss books about the chronic, awful boredom of an overeater's life. When we become obsessed with food, we can shut out everything and everyone.

It's boring to spend time hiding in the bathroom because you've hidden candy bars in the hamper.

It's boring to explain for the tenth time that your new diet will take time to show results.

It's boring to be scared to death of the medical clinic scale, the look on the nurse's face, and the disappointment in your doctor's eyes.

Overeating created a continuing crisis in our life, but today we have a program of healthy eating, exercise, and positive attitude that brings us more excitement than overeating ever could.

Today, see how exciting your life has become now that you play life to win.

*Today's Action Plan: I will never return to the awful boredom of living to eat.*

## October 15                    You Are Free to Choose

*Man's last freedom is his freedom to choose.*
*—Viktor Frankl*

You don't have to live in an underprivileged country or in a big-city ghetto to have a poor quality of life. Overeaters know they can make a food prison out of a mansion.

When you embraced your action plan, you created a comfort zone for yourself. That is why it is important that you learn to make changes whenever necessary to ensure continued healthy eating.

Taking charge of your life is a process of making choices and discovering what works for you. This is the continuing, exciting challenge of your life. In the end, all choice is yours, all responsibility, all victory.

Today, add a fresh appreciation for the rich diversity of choices you can make for your life. This is a freedom you've always wanted.

*Today's Action Plan: I will take charge of the quality of my life. Through good choices, I will make a palace of my prison.*

## October 16                    The Big Put-Off

*Often greater risk is involved in postponement than in making a wrong decision.*
*—H. A. Hopf*

"I'm going to stop overeating, and this time I really mean it!" Sounds final, doesn't it?

But what happens when, despite your vow, you overeat in the middle of the morning? After you overeat, you berate yourself. Instead of making a new beginning right on the spot, you postpone. "No sense starting over today. I already blew the diet, didn't I?"

So you spend the day overeating, using food to cover up your dislike for what you did. Next morning, you assure yourself you won't procrastinate again. Days and weeks, months and years pass in a blur of such broken promises, food binges, and tearful regrets.

Had enough of times like those? You bet you have! You can take action to get out of that hell. Now you have a direction and a plan in your life. You're a winner.

Today, decide that you will never again only vow to stop overeating. Trade broken vows for action.

*Today's Action Plan: I will not play a losing game with procrastination. I will play life to win.*

## October 17                    The Game of Pretend

*At last, I can be myself. I don't have to make things look good on the outside while I'm dying on the inside.*
*—Diet workshop participant*

Overeaters living in a thin society usually play three roles. The *happy clown* role says, "Everything's wonderful!" The *sad clown* role says, "Pity me!" The *flippant clown* role says, "I don't care!" Overweight people play so many roles they lose their real selves.

Did you try to make things look good on the outside, while feeling bad on the inside? Did you manipulate others to make them feel sorry for you? Or did you build an "I don't care" image and behave as if you believed it? Did you often wonder if overeating was worth it?

Now that you have a new lifestyle, you know that overeating is *not* worth it! You become who you truly are when you stop overeating, when you follow your healthy eating, exercise, and action plan. You like the new, honest, guilt-free person you have become.

Today, put away your repertoire of clown roles. Let the real you come through.

*Today's Action Plan: I will bring the curtain down on all false self-images. I will begin to find my true self.*

## October 18                                      Growing

*The more we can control our anxiety and reduce its crippling effects, the more we can make positive use of it in our striving to understand, accept, tolerate, and respect ourselves and others.*

*Henry Clay Lindgren*

A basic law of nature is that living things strive against all odds to grow. Growing, making positive changes, is healthy. When you overeat, you are in conflict with life's physical law of healthful growth. Excess food is an obstacle you can't get over or around on the way to fulfilling your potential.

Overeating must be eliminated before you can reach emotional maturity, and maturity is only one of the pleasures of growth; others are low anxiety, enhanced talents, and satisfying relationships.

Today, welcome the idea of positive change, so you can grow toward your full potential.

*Today's Action Plan: I will rid myself of excess food so I can be all I was meant to be. I will continue to grow emotionally.*

*Every one to whom much is given, of him much will be required.*

*—Luke 12:48*

Many overeaters struggling with food compulsion can barely tolerate themselves. It's unfortunate, because we've been given so much.

We've been given brains for clear thinking and wise judgment. But excess food dims our ability to think positively.

We've been given courage and strength to withstand living in a rapidly changing world. But overeating keeps us from using our courageous spirit.

We've been given heightened senses that can become blurred by bingeing.

We have all it takes to reach success. Only one obstacle stands in our way—overeating.

Today, make wise eating and exercise decisions, and power yourself into action. Now you are using what you have been given to make wonderful changes.

Today, use the wonderful abilities you've been given to make a winning change in your life.

*Today's Action Plan: I will use the abilities I've been given. I will get rid of the one obstacle that stands in my way—overeating.*

*As one thinketh in his heart, so is he.*

*—Proverbs 23:7*

Get quiet. At least once a day go to a place where you can hear the silence, where you will be able to listen to your inner voices without any distractions.

Understanding who you are, getting to know your own wants, demands time and the proper atmosphere for reflection. You don't have to go to a mountain top or a deserted beach, but it will help to get as far from interference as possible.

A quiet walk, a few minutes of solitude, a momentary vacation in a tranquil corner will give you a much-needed respite from the tension of life. Winners must rest and listen to their minds and bodies.

Today, grant yourself the peace of a few minutes out of your hectic day. Getting away from it all is one way you maintain a high performance level.

*Today's Action Plan: I will give myself a few minutes of my time. I will concentrate on my unique worth.*

## October 21                    Worst-Case Scenario

*There are days when it takes all you've got just to keep up.*

*—Robert Orben*

Some days you're faced with puzzling choices. Should you take this job or that one; move to the country or stay in the city? Those are the diet days when you're tempted to say, "Oh, the heck with it." At times like this it's easy to slip back into the practice of using food to deal with indecision.

Try using a worst-case scenario to help you decide. If you take the new job or move to the country, what's the worst thing that could happen? You could lose money or hate the country. Then what's the worst thing? You could get a new job or try to move back to your old neighborhood.

When you've made a bad choice, the worst thing that can happen is that you'll be faced with more choices.

But each time you choose, you learn.

Choice is only possible if you are in control of your eating. One of the hidden consequences of overeating is that you lose your decision-making abilities.

Today may begin with puzzling choices, but if you act rather than eat, you won't be at the mercy of happenstance.

*Today's Action Plan: I will not be trapped into overeating by indecision. I will be in charge of my choices.*

**October 22**                    **Double Reward**

*The effects of our actions may be postponed but they are never lost.*

—*Wu Ming Fu*

*Do today what you know you want to do.* This is a deceptively simple message that is life-saving. It tells us that when we don't do what we need and want to do, we come into immediate conflict with our own conscience.

There is a double reward for doing what you know you need to do. First, you feel worthwhile, not in conflict with your basic belief. Second, the job gets done. For overeaters this means building self-esteem and losing excess weight too.

Don't grab for the momentary pleasure of overeating, but reach for deeper rewards. Don't settle for the moment's indulgence when you can wait and have the double reward of self-esteem and a thinner, healthier body.

Today, do what you know you need to do for your body, mind, and emotions.

*Today's Action Plan: I will grab for real future rewards rather than a momentary food indulgence.*

## October 23

*Start again at your beginnings and never breathe a word about your loss.*
*—Rudyard Kipling*

Remember that time you lost a lot of weight? You were filled with joy. Life would be different—better, you thought. You would never again be overweight. But you got careless; action disappeared from your days, and the pounds came back fast.

Now again, you say, "This time when I lose weight, I won't forget how I did it." But you will, unless you and the principles of action are one, unless they become part of you and you become part of them. Keep doing what produced results.

Build discipline into your life. Some believe that discipline inhibits personal freedom, dries up creativity, and smothers spontaneity; but for overeaters it's a lifesaver. You need structure in your life.

Today, recognize the trap in forgetting your action plan. Don't change what works!

*Today's Action Plan: I will build structure into my life. I will take hold of the action principles and never let them go.*

## October 24 The Magic Hand from the Past

*More powerful is he who has himself in his own power.*
*—Lucius Annaeus Seneca*

Did your mother make you clean your plate? And does your mate complain about waste? And do your friends tempt you with fresh-baked goodies? No wonder you're overweight. It's all their fault!

It can be satisfying to blame others, but it's an irresponsible way to live. Fat is not something other people do to you. No matter what your mother told you as a child, as an adult you're making your own choices. There is no magic hand from the past controlling your fork.

Haven't you suffered long enough from the "magic hand"? Take charge of your life and the food in your life. It is the only way.

Today, see that the blame game is one you can't win. Take responsibility for your own eating. Take action.

*Today's Action Plan: I will take charge of the food in my life. I will be an achieving adult, not a victim.*

## October 25 See Success

*To try and to fail is at least to learn; to fail to try is to suffer the inestimable loss of what might have been.*
*—Chester Barnard*

Eating something not on your healthy eating plan doesn't mean you've lost everything. If you have been eating right for a week—for twenty-one meals—and you overate at one meal, you didn't blow the whole week. See the successes you had, and you will not lose perspective on that single overeating episode.

If you've set a weight goal and haven't reached it yet, don't see yourself as a failure. Accept your humanness. Saints don't make mistakes, but humans do.

Your way is no longer the all-or-nothing way of the frantic overeater or the frantic dieter. When you choose a positive, balanced perspective where successes are recognized, a stumble is something to learn from.

Today, see success as easily as you see failure. Accept

your humanness. This is the positive way you choose to live your life today and every day.

*Today's Action Plan: I will not let one stumble make me fall. I will achieve balance through a positive perspective.*

## October 26                                    Opportunities

*We consume our tomorrows fretting about our yesterdays.*

*—Persius*

To fret over wasted opportunity means that two opportunities—yesterday's and today's—have been wasted. Use today to get ahead of yesterday. Be too busy living, achieving, and planning to worry about yesterday's mistakes.

A person is really living when he or she can say, "I love where I am this minute, and I will love where I'm going to be tomorrow." What an optimistic, open, winning attitude!

Be a person who makes and then seizes opportunity. Be a winner who cares about good health, sticks to your eating plan, and keeps exercising your body. You'll notice the difference in how you feel about yourself, your life, and other people.

Today, stop fretting over yesterday's lost opportunities. You have become a winner who seizes opportunity.

*Today's Action Plan: I will forget yesterday's lost opportunities. I will seize today's chances and love every minute of it.*

*Behavior change is not easy—in fact it's damned hard—but it is possible. That thought's important to me after so many years of feeling helpless about my eating.*

> *—Man at a behavior-modification workshop*

Breaking an overeating habit isn't easy. During an ordinary day, many places, activities, and emotions cue you to eat. But habit, however strong, is curable.

Begin by developing a desirable, positive program. It's not too late to change the emotional habits that trigger overeating, nor is it too late to develop an exercise habit where none existed. To help you attain these ends,

1. Know that you can replace negative habits with positive new habits.

2. Never scold yourself for having an overeating problem. Instead, praise yourself for working hard to change your life.

3. Give yourself enough time to break a habit. How many years have you been overeating? You deserve as much time to make confirmed changes.

Today, take charge of your habits. What a positive step!

*Today's Action Plan: I will work at undoing my destructive habits. I know I can.*

*It's a pretty corrupt field.*

> *—Dr. William Bennett*

In the United States alone, it is estimated that billions of dollars are spent each year on fad dieting and the books, pills, and gadgets that go with it.

Most fad diets are nutritionally unbalanced, particularly single-food diets, from brown rice to grapefruit. And so far, no drug has been discovered that melts fat, blocks starch, or stops food cravings that come from the mind.

The blatant swindles come and go fast, but never disappear from the market. The product name changes, the spiel is updated, and the come-on ads are right back in the media.

But the only real miracle ingredient is you. When you take charge of your life, when you become the director of your own action, no pill, magic food, or diet-marketeer can do what you can do.

Today, reject the attempts to capitalize on your misery. Fat is not forever, because you won't allow it.

*Today's Action Plan: I will not be mesmerized by promises of diet magic. I will make my own miracle.*

## October 29                                    Get the Fat Out

*Get the fat in your diet to be less than 30 percent of the calories you take in, and everything else falls into line.*

*—Dr. George H. Blackburn*

To develop a personal right-eating plan, it's best to work with a nutritionist or educate yourself through nutrition books. A good nutritionist or text will help you adjust your diet to include a mixture of protein, carbohydrates, and most important, 30 percent (many scientists recommend 20 percent) of total fat.

You will want your diet to:
1. Provide a balance of essential vitamins and minerals
2. Furnish ample food fibers
3. Deliver weight-loss and weight-control

4. Fit your way of living
5. Bring you to optimum health

By learning about what you need to eat, you're taking charge of your life.

Today, take charge of the food in your life; be aware of the protein, fat, and carbohydrates in your diet.

*Today's Action Plan: I will be in charge of my own right-eating plan. When I need nutritional help, I will get it.*

## October 30                              Weight Slaves

*When I weighed 239 pounds, I thought I had no right to be seen on the street, to eat in a restaurant, to live!*
*—Woman at a diet group*

You are a person with all the rights to live that other people have. Your weight, whatever it is, doesn't change that basic fact.

*Carry yourself like a winner everywhere you go.* Watch people of all sizes. You'll easily be able to separate life's winners from the walking apologies. The apologists have their shoulders hunched and look at the ground, hoping no one will notice them. Winners walk with heads high, eyes curious about the world. Their confident bearing declares: "I'm a beautiful person!"

Many overweight people have been ridiculed, ostracized, and laughed at. But winners believe in their rights as humans. There's only one right you don't have: the right to retreat into apathy and self-pity.

Today, carry yourself like a winner. You have rejected weight-slavery.

*Today's Action Plan: I will carry a sign that says, "I'm a beautiful human being." I will never give up my rights.*

*He that resolves upon any great and good end has, by that very resolution, scaled the chief barrier to it.*
—*Tryon Edwards*

Let's say you're applying for work you really want—the job of losing weight and changing your life. Now make a mental resumé listing your qualifications. You wouldn't begin by criticizing yourself: "I'm a stupid, rotten person who can't even control food."

Clean up your personal resumé. If you wrote any negative statements like the one above, delete them. They disqualify you for the success you seek. Concentrate instead on your positive ideas and get into action.

You are capable of getting the most out of new experiences. The world will make way for people like you. But first, you must become the person you want to be: through healthy eating, exercise, and a self-accepting view of yourself.

Today, clean out all the negative garbage from your "life resumé."

*Today's Action Plan: I will not disqualify myself for the job of living a thin and healthy life. I will get out into the world and live.*

**November 1**                           **For the Health of It**

*Lethargy does not make fat; fat makes lethargy.*
> *—Anonymous*

Sedentary people don't always gain weight, but over-weight people are often sedentary. We tend to focus on activities that aren't very physical. We especially want to avoid the embarrassment of exercising in public. But we pay a high price for physical unfitness.

Exercise helps you lose weight faster and healthier, reduces your appetite, increases your sense of emotional well-being, and improves your muscle and skin tone. But most of all, it gives you the sense of owning your own body.

Few people give regular exercise the six to eight weeks it takes to experience real changes. Be one of the few who does and enjoy the results.

Today, choose the benefits over the difficulties of exercise. Make the commitment to overall health.

*Today's Action Plan: I will give myself time to achieve body changes. I will see that looking and feeling great was worth the effort.*

**November 2**                                **Junk Thinking**

*I don't care to belong to any club that will accept me for a member.*
> *—Groucho Marx*

Most overweight people feel they aren't worth the effort it takes to lose weight. That's why their diets often fail and they regain any weight they've lost. Then they push away others' affection, thinking, "If people love me, they must be losers." This destroys their self-image and possibility for success.

Take the self-hate out of weight loss. You are learning that your feelings are only a starting point. They must be followed by commitment to action. Only time and plain hard work bring about change.

Use your action skills to put more self-esteem into your self-image. If others love you, they must be winners.

Today, realize that rejecting others because you thought yourself unworthy was junk thinking.

*Today's Action Plan: I will remember that I am worthy of good things. I will use my action skills today.*

**November 3**                    **Create a Commercial**

*The grand essentials to happiness in this life are something to do, something to love, and something to hope for.*

—*Joseph Addison*

You must come to understand that you are unique. One way you can illustrate this idea to yourself is to imagine yourself as the star of your own commercial.

To build self-confidence, particularly before facing a tough day, try reciting a short personal commercial with an "I look good, I feel fine" message.

Your own special commercial can go something like this:

> *As long as there's (your name), there's action, reliability, and excellence. (Your name) stands for the best in healthy*

> *eating, physical fitness, and a winning
> view of life. To top it off, you get 24-
> hour commitment, 365 days a year.
> Believe in (your name) today!*

Today, sell yourself on your own commercial, a pep talk for extra confidence.

> *Today's Action Plan: I will use my commercial when I need a mental boost. I will endorse my own pro-duct—me.*

## November 4         The Shape of Things to Come

> *We wish to be happier than other people, and this is always difficult, for we believe others to be happier than they are.*
>
> *—Baron de Montesquieu*

If you idealize thin people, think again. Their lives aren't always models of satisfaction. They may not have our health problems, but being thin does not banish all troubles.

Some overeaters feel cheated when they lose weight and find their lives aren't perfect. Situations at home and at work will always require give-and-take, no matter what your weight is. Others expect you to handle problems just like everyone else.

But being thin and healthy will have its advantages: you will have a more attractive, energetic body to live in and a new lifestyle that shows you how to aim at goals and win.

Today, take a realistic look at thinness.

> *Today's Action Plan: I will prepare myself by under-standing that a thinner me won't be problem-free.*

*The person who can laugh with life has developed deep roots with confidence and faith—faith in oneself, in people and in the world, as contrasted to negative ideas with distrust and discouragement.*

*—Democritus*

The sixth principle in your action plan tells you to make your own sunlight. We overweight people have more than our share of burdens. Learning to relax and laugh is a link with the good life.

Laughter demolishes anger. That's why we sometimes resist laughing when we're upset; self-righteously we want to hang on to the drama a bit longer.

Laughter doesn't land on our doorstep. We must create it ourselves from our hope and determination to make our lives work better. Leave time for fun and laughter. Be a sunshine-maker, and every good laugh will be a minivacation in the midst of your day.

Today, smile and laugh with a winner's gusto.

*Today's Action Plan: I will let go of burdens and embrace laughter often today.*

*The most exhausting thing in life is being insincere.*
*—Anne Morrow Lindbergh*

You know you have talent, ambition, and strength. But how do you become who you really are?

Begin by removing yourself from diet talk. All the what-I-ate-yesterday histories—"foodalogs"—tend to define you as only a food machine.

Lead a well-rounded life. High achievers have a variety of relationships and interests other than food. They pay attention to their spiritual and emotional growth too.

Seek direction rather than perfection. Your weight today is less important than the direction you're going. Is your weight going down or has it stabilized? Do you feel great? These are results you want.

Compete with yourself, not others. True champions enjoy improving their own performance more than beating their competitors. A winner is not self-defeating.

Today, choose to lead a well-rounded life, to seek direction, and to compete only with yourself.

*Today's Action Plan: I will be who I am, not what I think others expect. I will practice a winner's skills.*

### November 7          Are You Eating Too Much Fat?

*It almost seems as if there's a conspiracy to keep our fat intake excessive.*

*—Carol Flinders*

Processed food, restaurant cooking, and most snack foods are usually high in saturated fats. As a result, the diet most people follow—thin or fat—contains at least 35 percent fat. This is a priority problem for you since your weight-loss eating plan should have between 20 and 30 percent fat.

Learn to read labels. A gram of fat has nine calories. If the meal has twelve grams (108 calories) of fat in a total of 400 calories, then it's 25 percent fat—about right for your eating plan. On the other hand, based on the same measurement, you'll find that mayonnaise contains about 90 percent fat—definitely not recommended for your eating plan.

Today, take control of the fat in your food. When you do, you'll enjoy better health and appearance.

*Today's Action Plan: I will reduce the fat content of my food.*

---

**November 8**         **A Fast-Acting Cure for the Blues**

*Knowledge is not power. Action, which is knowledge in motion, does the work of the world.*
*—Walter A. Heiby*

When you know you need to eat less, but you continue to overeat and gain weight, you endure incredible turmoil.

To quiet the tempest, return to a simple idea: "I will act out my desire for a new lifestyle." With such a philosophy, conflict is removed and depression is banished. It takes only a few minutes to make the basic decision to eat right today. After that, move away from preoccupation with food.

The whole point of your new lifestyle is not merely to exchange an eating machine for a dieting machine. You've got more important things to do and successes to achieve. The rest of your life beckons you on.

Today, see that the fastest cure for depression is erasing the conflict between what you want for your life and what you are actually doing.

*Today's Action Plan: I will act upon my desire for a new life with style. I will become part of the big world outside of my weight problem.*

---

**November 9**         **Reject Unfairness and Seek Support**

*All of the art of living lies in a fine mingling of letting go and holding on.*
*—Havelock Ellis*

A bystander laughs at you while you're taking a brisk

walk in your neighborhood. A nurse scolds you because your weight goal doesn't correspond with her charts. An acquaintance demeans your success. Such slights aren't fair!

Unfair things have happened to you before and may happen again. But it's not because you deserve to be treated cruelly.

Unfair people often have bigger problems than you do, unless you make their problems yours. And you do that if you carry around their image of you, rather than your own.

Reject their unfairness. Learn to seek and accept the good, kind, supportive people you know. Let go of the idea that fat makes you unworthy of love and acceptance. Hold on to what you are becoming through your healthy eating, energizing lifestyle.

People are sometimes unfair, but it's their problem. Today, you refuse to make their problem your problem.

*Today's Action Plan: I reject the unfairness of others. I will win no matter what others say or do.*

## November 10                    Think on These Things

*We think too small—like the frog at the bottom of the well. He thinks the sky is only as big as the top of the well. If he surfaced, he would have an entirely different view.*

—Mao Tse-tung

There are five major themes running through this book that can build a strong foundation for your new lifestyle if you come to know them well:

1. Your conflict and unhappiness decrease in direct proportion to the inner harmony you achieve.

2. You are capable as you are, and you have everything you need to become a winner.

3. Action creates motivations, not the other way around.

4. Action is a precondition for increasing your self-esteem.

5. You make your own choices. Others have power over you only if you choose to grant it.

Repeat these powerful themes, and use them every day when the going gets tough. They'll keep you strong.

Today "see the whole sky." Commit yourself to applying the themes of this book to your new life.

*Today's Action Plan: I will learn these power-filled themes. When the going gets tough, I will use them for strength.*

**November 11**     **Exercise for the Person Too Busy to Exercise**

*After my husband's heart attack, the doctor prescribed two miles of brisk walking. If walking is that good for him, I figured it would be great for me.*
*—Diet center speaker*

You're a busy person in a fast-moving world—how can you fit in regular exercise? Consider the perfect exercise for too-busy people: walking. It fits into small time periods, and unlike running, swimming, or tennis, it requires no special clothes, or places, or even a shower afterward.

Walk every chance you get—to and from work or shopping, if that's possible. Take a walk during your lunch hour. See how many city blocks you can cover in fifteen or thirty minutes. Even a short walk each day will make a difference.

Walking's natural rhythm has a relaxing quality, and it tones your muscles, expands your lung capacity, helps weight loss, reduces fatigue, and makes you feel younger.

Today, take a walk. It fits neatly into any busy schedule.

*Today's Action Plan: I will walk whenever I get a few minutes. I will reap many benefits from this most convenient form of exercise.*

**November 12**                    **Your Margin of Tranquillity**

*Without a certain margin of tranquillity, truth succumbs.*

—*José Ortega y Gasset*

When you were overeating, did you deliberately remove pleasure from your life? Did you say, "If I'm fat, I don't deserve to have fun"?

Now that you have taken charge of your overeating, energized your body, and adopted a positive view, you have begun to create an emotional comfort zone around your life.

Avoid being in a frantic rush. You don't have to hurry to lose weight, hurry to meet the right mate, hurry to have fun.

Live all the days of your life, beginning with today. Relax. Take time for walking in the park, reading fine literature, or developing your inner spiritual life. Slow your frantic pace and experience the beauty around you, the pleasure of this moment. Isn't it wonderful to inject some tranquility?

Today, put pleasure back into your life. You have created an emotional comfort zone of right-eating and right-thinking.

*Today's Action Plan: I will put pleasure into this day. I will add tranquillity to my emotional life.*

*A fellow doesn't last long on what he has done. He's got to keep delivering as he goes along.*
                                        —*Carl Hubbell*

Years of studies about motivation have concluded that flashy initial success doesn't always predict long-term performance. The most reliable predictor of success is commitment.

Commitment is a fire fueled by persistence. You develop a burning passion to pursue your goal and continually feed the flame of self-confidence with small, interim goals along the way.

Achievement-oriented people never stagnate. They learn constantly, adding to their knowledge every day. When you ask yourself each day: "What will I learn today?" you won't dissipate time and energy in aimless activity.

You have numerous learning opportunities that will make a difference in your life. Learn about nutrition, about your body and mind, and about the beautiful world you live in. When you do, you will keep moving toward your goals.

Today, commit your life to the living goals you set for yourself.

*Today's Action Plan: I will renew my commitment to the winning life and keep on delivering it every day.*

*Facing a task of this magnitude requires fortitude, dedication and motivation. The patient must not be made to feel like a glutton or sinner.*
—The Merck Manual of Diagnosis and Therapy

You weren't born overweight, and you might not have been overweight as a child or adolescent. But sometime in your life you changed from eating-to-live to living-to-eat.

You probably first overate to help deal with stress. Soon your binges became more frequent, even planned. Eventually you overate when you felt good *or* bad.

Food became a payoff for enduring frustrations and coping with daily stress. Finally, you no longer linked eating with pleasure or pain. All emotions caused cravings.

To control your overeating, you must sever your emotional bond to food and make new emotional connections to success, to your body, and to your attitudes. With your new, positive self-concept, you have the courage to do so.

Today, you have discovered the nature of an overeater's addiction. What you once learned about food can be relearned.

*Today's Action Plan: I will build new emotional connections omitting food.*


**November 15**                    **The Loneliness of a**
                                   **Longtime Overeater**

*Loneliness is the fear of love.*

                                   —*Ira Tanner*

It's easy to feel alone in today's world. We live in impersonal big cities or behind suburbia's fences. We leave families and friends to move far away. But being alone is not the same as loneliness—feeling disconnected from others and even ourselves.

When you overeat, you feel your loneliness inside, but what's worse, you believe you deserve to be lonely.

You may think you are worthless.

Around others, you focus on your own feelings, reading negativity into other people's minds. It's difficult to project an open-for-friendship attitude when you are so self-focused. To start a friendship, you must consider the feelings of others as well as your own.

If you stick to it, your new lifestyle will give you confidence and increased self-esteem. You will begin to do wonderful things, and your action-taking attitudes will start to show.

Today, decide to defeat loneliness by projecting an open-for-friendship attitude.

*Today's Action Plan: I will be a friend to myself so that I can be a friend to others.*

**November 16**                    **Your Working Dream**

*We shall become what we wish to become, do what we wish to do, when our habitual thought corresponds with our desire.*

*—Orison Swett Marden*

We see an endless stream of drastic commercial diet regimens—eating one fruit, taking one powder, drinking one liquid. Medicine offers equally drastic remedies—bypass operations, jaw-wiring, and stomach-stapling. But these methods don't deal with overeaters' minds.

Most of these remedies treat overeaters as passive objects for manipulation rather than active participants in their own recovery. The idea that you have the right and the ability to take charge of your life, to become a self-manager, may be discounted or ignored.

Through your action plan, you have made your mind a powerful resource for changing your body. Thus you have become focused on your dream of a healthier lifestyle. Even more important, because you are taking action, you make your dream a working dream.

Today, see that you have more power over your life than ever before.

*Today's Action Plan: I will become a self-manager. I will be an active participant in my recovery from overeating.*

**November 17**                    **Your Mind Matters**

*The used key is always bright.*
                    —*Benjamin Franklin*

Thoughts are real and powerful. Look at what you've accomplished through the power of thought. You have become what you are with the strength of your mind.

You have control over your own thoughts, and you control what you do about them. Most important, your mind can control your overeating problem.

When you apply mind-solutions to your problem, you are authorizing yourself to create control for overeating. You give permission to work from the inside out, not from the outside in.

In the past, you did not control overeating because of what others thought or said, and you weren't helped by outside controls that dictated you should lose weight.

Today, know that your thoughts are what will change the circumstances of your life. The decision to take charge of what you eat is a tangible event you made happen.

*Today's Action Plan: I will connect my mind to my overeating problem. I will become what my own thoughts direct me to be.*

*Since the early 1900s Americans have actually decreased their food intake, become more sedentary, and grown fatter. It's clear that the problem is not eating too much, but exercising too little.*

—Dr. Peter Wood

Great-grandmother fed the chickens, made two trips to the root cellar, and pumped well water for washday all before 8 a.m. Great-grandfather chopped wood, brought in the cows from pasture, milked and fed them—all before breakfast. What would they think of today's automated society?

For years, overweight has been charged to gluttony. Of course overeating occurs. But it is erroneous to ignore the major contributor to today's weight problem: lack of energy expenditure.

Perhaps we can take a few tips from our forebears. We can easily add exercise to our daily routines by substituting physical tasks for automated ones—*getting up* and turning off the TV, for example, then taking a short walk or climbing some stairs while we're up.

Today, get on the weight-losing track by finding new tasks that can double as exercise.

*Today's Action Plan: I will discard automated thinking. I will find tasks that can double as exercises.*

**November 19**                              **Expect Victory**

*Lack of faith in yourself, in what life will do for you, cuts you off from the good things of the world. Expect victory and you make victory.*

—Preston Bradley

"Believe in yourself" isn't just a bumper-sticker phrase. It's a practical tool. One season, the underdog Notre Dame basketball team had to face undefeated UCLA, a team with the longest winning streak in basketball history. On the day before the big game, the Notre Dame coach gave his team a special drill. He had them practice cutting the net off the hoop—a victory ritual. To everyone's surprise, Notre Dame won the contest by one point, and the champions snipped away the net just as they had rehearsed.

Having faith in your success doesn't mean you sit back and wait for somebody to hand it to you—you have to plant yourself firmly in front of destiny. Prepare yourself for victory with healthy eating, exercise, and winning attitudes.

Today, adopt an expectation of victory and prepare yourself to receive success.

*Today's Action Plan: I will prepare to win. I will expect victory and accept nothing less.*

**November 20**                    **Planners Succeed**

*Success is planned for and planners have success.*
                                        —*Larry Worman*

Overeating brings chaos, yet we tend to shy away from putting structure into our lives. Structure often looks like too much trouble, so we procrastinate. But when we make the effort to replace chaos with structure, we realize just how beautiful life can be.

Spend a few minutes planning for success. You know the formula by now: set goals, make a commitment, take action, keep motivating yourself.

Motivation comes from two places. Outside rewards are one source, but the most lasting motivation comes from the confidence that "I'm doing this because I want to, not because I have to."

This certainty that you are worthy of your best efforts puts you in control of your thinking—and of your planning. And planners succeed.

Today, plan for success. This is the only life you have, and you want to make it a beautiful one.

*Today's Action Plan: I will not postpone plans for my life. I will plan because I want to, not because I have to.*

### November 21                    Worry Is Not Responsibility

*Worry is a thin stream of fear trickling through the mind. If encouraged, it cuts a channel into which all other thoughts are drained.*
*—Arthur Somers Roche*

There's a story about a man who was so worried about elephants that he burned incense constantly to keep them away. "Nonsense," said a friend, "there are absolutely no elephants in this country." Replied the worrier, "See? My incense is working."

The same is true for overeaters; worrying about overeating doesn't work. Rather than warding off the problem, worry actually gives it life. When you worry instead of taking positive action, you think negative thoughts, push out positive ones, and set yourself up for failure.

Worry takes valuable time—time you need to take action on your real problems. It's a clever device your inner negative critic uses to keep you inactive. But if you learn to plan actively for a positive future, you'll feel more in control. Your critic can't manage an optimist like you.

Today, worry less about elephants and take action on your real problems.

*Today's Action Plan: I will decide what I want to change, and then do it, instead of just worrying about it.*

**November 22**                              **No One Is Born to Fail**

*The whole philosophy of failure can be summed up in three words, "What's the use?"*

*—Anonymous*

One of the greatest moments in your life will come when you realize that you were born to succeed, not fail. On that day, you'll have a feeling of wholeness, identity, and continuity with yourself that you can depend on for life. From that moment, you will be good company for yourself.

Hasten that day by telling yourself, "I am smart, I am strong, and I am in control." This will help you to see the person you really are.

Winners are people who take charge, who let nothing negative interfere with their plans. Taking charge of their lives becomes a series of positive actions. "What's the use?" is a defeatist phrase that has no place in their vocabulary—or yours.

Today, begin working for the greatest day of your life—the day when you'll know that you are whole.

*Today's Action Plan: I will be a winner. I will never ask, "What's the use?"*

*Overzealous beginners start out too quickly and intensely with their program, and wind up burning out mentally or else placing too much stress on not-yet-well-developed muscles.*

            *—Dr. Jesse DeLee*

We all-or-nothing people are apt to start an exercise program too fast, go too far, and become disillusioned about exercise.

It is particularly important that overweight exercisers begin slowly but steadily. If you want to run, start by walking, then move to a jog. If you find running too hard on your feet or joints, pull back to a walk. You'll still get weight-loss benefit, because without injuries, you'll be able to stick to it.

And sticking with regular exercise gives your life structure. When you program exercise into your day, your other activities must be better organized to make them all fit.

Start slowly, build your endurance and skill, pull back when necessary—but keep at it.

Today, heed to the old proverb: Slow and steady wins the race.

*Today's Action Plan: I will aim for total fitness. I will exercise like a winner.*

*Unless there be correct thought, there cannot be any action, and when there is correct thought, right action will follow.*

            *—Henry George*

Working with our action plans every day means we

deal with realities. We are discovering within ourselves the capacity to take charge of our thoughts, bodies, and affairs. We painfully realize we could have done much more much sooner, but when we thought we were limited, we saw no point in striving. Now, as our capabilities open to us, we must deal with our newfound potential.

How do you do this? Begin by remembering how you learned new games as a child. You couldn't keep up at first, but you knew you should keep trying. Did you work until you mastered the game, or did you walk away saying, "That was a dumb game, anyway"?

In the process of becoming all that you can be, you will be greatly challenged. You can call these challenges "dumb" and walk away, or you can keep trying and give the game of life the best you've got.

Today, see that the pain of knowing is discovering the glorious potential that lies hidden inside you.

*Today's Action Plan: I will play every game up to my potential. I will keep trying.*

## November 25          Exercise Your Self-Esteem

*You come into the world with nothing, and the purpose of your life is to make something out of nothing.*
*—H. L. Mencken*

There probably isn't one idea in this book that you weren't already aware of on some level. You might even have told yourself some of the same things you read. However, you didn't follow your own good advice.

Today when you promise yourself you're going to lose weight, you'll follow through. You won't make a promise that you have no intention of keeping.

Take the time today to complete one simple task

you've been avoiding. This will increase your self-esteem. Suppose you fall down today. Don't become too discouraged to take the next risk. Focus your attention on getting up and beginning again.

Today, be reasonable with yourself. Less will overwhelm you, and you will be encouraged to reach for your goals.

*Today's Action Plan: I will listen to my own good advice. I will exercise my self-esteem so that I will be receptive to good ideas.*

**November 26**                    **Exercise—A Natural Therapy**

*Tension is trapped energy.*
                              *—Naura Hayden*

Tension is a familiar feeling for most overeaters. We can thank it for many of our extra pounds. One way to manage tension is to treat it as trapped energy that can be released daily through physical exercise.

Imagine your tension as energy bursting to get out. Now think of play, movement, and exercise as energy safety valves allowing you to dissipate tension while losing weight and toning your body. You'll find there are few things in this world with so many benefits wrapped up in a few minutes of daily commitment.

Get moving today. A half-hour walk is heaven compared to a half-hour food binge. Likewise, your stationary bicycle is far better for you than a battle with your boss, mate, or neighbor.

Today, release your tension-energy the winning way, with exercise.

*Today's Action Plan: I will not overeat because of tension. I will exercise my nerves instead.*

*I think everyone's second business is their occupation
and their first business is to know themselves.*
                                    *—Jo Coudert*

A strange inner struggle wages inside most overeaters.
One part of us is defiant and says, "I don't want to eat
less and exercise more!" But the other part shouts,
"Somebody, *please,* help me stop!" How can both these
thoughts coexist in one brain?

Imagine two chairs facing each other—your "help-
me" self in one chair, your "defiant" self seated opposite. Now let "defiant" scream how it hates knuckling
under to authority. Next have "help me" explain how
fighting structure has always gotten you in trouble, how
unhappy you are with overeating, and how you have
decided to change. "Defiant" may argue but can offer
no alternative to overeating.

Role-playing can be an effective way to demonstrate
how determined you are to not let anyone, including
yourself, get in the way of your new plan.

Today, play a mind game to help you sort out what
you really want.

*Today's Action Plan: I will not overeat out of defiance.
I will make it my business to know myself.*

*When you know who you are and you realize what
you can do, you can do things better at forty than
when you're twenty.*
                                    *—Shirley MacLaine*

Thinking of themselves as deprived children, unloved
and unlovable, is a real gut feeling for many overeaters.
It's not that they aren't lovable; they *feel* unloved.

To feel lovable, acknowledge the loving things you do for others. Have you visited a sick person, fixed a child's hurt, listened sympathetically to a friend's troubles?

Think of the lovable qualities you usually hide from others. Have you worked for or given to a charity, laughed aloud, or sung joyously? All these prove your lovability.

Today, give yourself loving attention and praise for all the kind, thoughtful, generous gifts you give to others. Accept the love and attention offered by the people who love you.

*Today's Action Plan: I will accept my loving and lovable qualities so that I will allow myself to deserve the happiness of food control.*

**November 29**                                    **Your Verbal Diary**

*It is the disease of not listening...that I am troubled withal.*

—*William Shakespeare*

Sometimes we think hiding our emotions keeps us safe, but it endangers us more than we know. To keep those feelings locked inside, we often smother them with food. Instead, we need to learn what we're feeling and act on it.

For the next week, set aside fifteen minutes at the end of each day. Tape-record or write down your thoughts and feelings about the day's events.

At the end of the week, play back your tape (or recite your written diary) and really hear what you've said to yourself. Pay attention to what you felt and how you expressed those feelings. Can you share them with someone close to you? Pick two or three appropriate feelings and express them to a trusted, sympathetic friend or relative. You've begun opening yourself to others.

Today, try sharing your feelings instead of stuffing them down with food.

*Today's Action Plan: I will start my verbal diary tonight. I will express my feelings so I won't have to smother them by overeating.*

**November 30**                    **The Three Rs of Friendship**

*What we see depends mainly on what we look for.*
                                        —*John Lubbock*

If you think you shouldn't burden your friends with your problems, you're ignoring a source of emotional support. Friendly support doesn't just make life easier for you, but it can keep your motivation high. And motivation is the lifeblood of your healthy eating, body energizing, and attitude-changing lifestyle.

Gain your friends' emotional support by following the three Rs:

1. *Reach out*—let your friends know you need them.

2. Pick the *right person* to share your emotional problem with, one who will be understanding.

3. Have *realistic expectations*—don't expect too much from your friends. A sympathetic ear is often enough.

When you share emotional problems with friends, you pay them the highest compliment. You show that you trust them and respect their judgment.

Today, use the three Rs to gain emotional support.

*Today's Action Plan: I will reach out for emotional support when I need it. I will be willing to share my problems to safeguard my healthy eating plan.*

## December 1              Where to Start and Stay

*To live is to change, and to be perfect is to have changed often.*

           *—John Henry Cardinal Newman*

If you've been overweight for some time, your weight probably is the central fact of your existence. It may affect your choice of work, your social roles, and your attitudes about yourself. You may see yourself as an outcast, helpless and hopeless. You may be caught in a vicious cycle of low self-esteem and overeating.

It's important to remember that you are a valid person regardless of your present size. That is a simple fact. But also remember the benefits of losing weight: you will probably live longer as a thinner person and enjoy improved health, looks, and energy. You will live in a real, if sometimes unfair, world instead of living in a make-believe world of overeating.

Today, decide to keep your self-esteem high and live comfortably in the real world.

*Today's Action Plan: I will accept my personal value. I will make a choice each day to remove food from the center of my existence.*

*Man is not what he thinks he is, but what he thinks,*
*he is.*
— *Elbert Hubbard*

Submerged defiance is a part of many overeaters'
makeups. It causes us to resist the kind of orderliness
that healthy eating and physical and mental fitness creates. You may think a structured way of life sounds too
oppressive, but as an overeater, you abide by certain
rules that are much more restrictive:

1. You cannot buy nice clothes, disagree with
friends, or believe compliments.

2. You can never enjoy food and must postpone living until you are thin.

3. You don't deserve satisfying relationships.

4. You can never say no to the demands of others.

5. You can never praise yourself or feel good about
anything you do.

Which set of rules will you follow, the overeater's
rules or your action principles? The freedom to overeat
carries with it the most restrictions, and your action
plan offers the most freedom.

Today, choose freedom from overeating.

*Today's Action Plan: I will follow the plan that allows*
*me maximum freedom.*

*There is very little difference in people, but that little*
*difference makes a big difference. The little difference*
*is attitude. The big difference is whether it is positive*
*or negative.*
— *W. Clement Stone*

A woman boarded an airplane enroute to a diet group convention. To her dismay, she was seated next to a man who was so obese that two seats and two belts had to be specially rigged to fit him. "I was so embarrassed," she recalled. "I didn't want others in the plane to identify me with this fat man. I knew that my animosity toward him was also directed at myself."

Some of us have so incorporated our society's disgust with fat, we actually dislike other overweight people—we project onto them what we don't like in ourselves. This attitude is a disguised self-punishment.

On the other hand, when we develop compassion for other overweight people, we have compassion for ourselves. And we need more compassion to allow ourselves to win.

Today, take responsibility for your attitude. Try to have compassion for others like you.

*Today's Action Plan: I will have compassion for myself so that I can know compassion for others. I will not punish myself by assimilating society's disgust for fat.*

### December 4                    Five Favorite Fat Alibis

*I like a state of continual becoming, with a goal in front and not behind.*

*—George Bernard Shaw*

Most of us who've had many diet setbacks had to find reasons for our failures: "Mother forced me to eat when I was young." "I can't throw food out; it's wasteful." "Everyone in my family is fat." "I'm so nervous, I can't stop eating."

When you adopt the winning attitudes of your action plan, you assume responsibility for your overeating and what it has done to your body and life. We can't go back and change our childhood or our genes. But we can change ourselves now, create realistic goals, and adopt the strategies that will take us to them.

Often, as a final excuse, we say, "I can't stand another diet!" Say instead: "I can't stand another day of overeating!"

Today, let go of all excuses for postponing your life. Adopt winning attitudes with goals.

*Today's Action Plan: I will reject excuses for failure. I will embrace self-responsibility for my overeating and take action.*

## December 5        You Can Help Yourself

*Why let luck decide?*

*—Gilbert Barnes*

The idea of using mind power to solve weight problems is tough to accept. But if you translate willpower into concepts such as self-reliance, strength of purpose, and faith in yourself, you can see that it can play a part in recovery.

It's tough to kick a food addiction by yourself; however, with strength of mind, you can add immeasurably to the help you get from support groups or professional help. You can triumph over food—if you believe you can.

You possess far more strength than you might think and strong-minded people believe, with everything they have, that they can do it. With that attitude, recovery is not only possible, but inevitable.

Today, see how determination, the power of your mind, and faith in yourself can help work miracles.

*Today's Action Plan: I will use my strength of will, whatever my diet plan. I will believe I can stop abusing food.*

**December 6**   **Good for the Body,**
**Good for the Mind**

*The idea is to keep moving. Even a little bit is better than none.*
*—Dr. Everett L. Smith*

It is well accepted that exercise increases endurance and muscle strength and decreases blood pressure and heart rate. But people are often surprised by the pleasant mental and emotional side effects of exercise.

At least once today, do enough extra moving to make your heart beat faster. You can do this by walking faster than normal, by dancing, or by practicing a good routine of calisthenics. The effects will last all day.

One great effect is that exercise will not make you hungrier—just the opposite—you'll want less to eat. This appetite suppressant costs nothing and works better than any drug, potion, or magic diet on the market.

Move more today and put more delight into your life. You have something that really works to reduce your appetite and weight.

*Today's Action Plan: I will incorporate exercise into my life today. I will move more and enjoy life more.*

**December 7**   **Your Greatest Discovery**

*Putting off an easy thing makes it difficult; putting off a hard one makes it impossible.*
*—George H. Lorimer*

The most important discovery of your life may be the

untapped power of your own mind. You can read books, hear lectures, or collect diplomas, but none of these scholarly pursuits can give you more power to change your life than you already possess.

Your power of thought rules your inner world. If you declare, "I feel awful," you will be sick today. But if you say, "I feel terrific!" then you will be empowered with healthy optimism.

Today your mind rules your destiny, forms your living environment, changes your personality. As you think negatively or positively, you harm or heal yourself. What freedom this gives you. Rather than being helpless at the hands of unseen, uncontrollable forces, you can make the necessary changes to meet the demands of your day.

Today, discover the power of your positive mind to change your destiny from food-dependence to food control.

*Today's Action Plan: I will use my thought power to take charge of overeating. I will make my own discovery.*

## December 8                                        Your Perfect Right

*Self-distrust is the cause of many of our failures.*
                                        —*Christian N. Bovee*

We overeaters often don't think we deserve the same rights as others. We become martyrs, unable to grant ourselves the slightest pleasure. This punishing and limiting attitude closes off pleasure, as well as potential solutions to our food problem.

You do have rights, the same as anyone:

• You have a perfect right to deny unreasonable requests —graciously, but always firmly.

- You have a perfect right to wear the clothes you like and to walk in the sun without a dark coat to hide under.
- You have a perfect right to exercise in public without harassment.
- You have a perfect right to use your talents at home, at work, or at a social gathering, no matter what you weigh.

If you catch yourself thinking, "I can't," counter back with, "Yes, I can, and I have a perfect right to do so." You have the right to be in control.

Today, you already have every right you need. Trust yourself.

*Today's Action Plan: I will not be a martyr to my weight. I will use my rights.*

**December 9**                    **Be Your Best Friend**

*Most people who engage in self-destructive behavior have simply chosen an ill-advised method of getting relief from the pain of their lives.*
                    —*Dr. John W. Bush*

You may see fate as the enemy that got you into your overeating mess. Can it be, though, that your worst enemy was you? Using food to cope with a problem unrelated to physical hunger was self-defeating. Food binges solved no problems, but created a new one—fat.

Now, find a mirror and look in it. The person you see there can be your best friend. Take one action to prove this friendship.

Tell your mirror image, "Today, I will work the action plan. I will do it for you." That's what a good friend would say.

Today, decide to be your own best friend, not your worst enemy. You're somebody you'd like to know.

*Today's Action Plan: Today I will cope by using my healthy eating plan, exercise, and positive attitude. I will send only positive messages to my best friend.*

## December 10        The Secret of Weight Maintenance

*Exercise is the great appetite equalizer.*

*—Anonymous*

Regular physical activity helps you stabilize your weight. Food portion control *is* important, but the secret to maintaining your weight after shedding pounds is to continue your exercise program. If your scales show your weight is up, increase your exercise.

When you arrive at your target weight, try expanding your exercise repertoire. Exercise boosts the self-discipline needed for weight maintenance. Your mind becomes focused, your thoughts concentrated, your energies channeled.

After exercising, you're in your own self-made world: physical energy spent, but mind clear and strengthened. Controlled eating then becomes just an extension of your physical and mental discipline.

Today, work on stabilizing your natural weight with exercise. The whole world of exercise is now open to you.

*Today's Action Plan: If my weight is above my comfortable level, I will exercise longer.*

## December 11        The Special Person Inside You

*Don't bother just to be better than your contemporaries or predecessors. Try to be better than yourself.*

*—William Faulkner*

There is a special person inside you—a good, energetic, achieving person. That person was kept prisoner, condemned to unhappiness as long as you indulged in anger, guilt, and self-ridicule.

Now, you have the ability to think yourself through your overeating and living problems. You don't need special equipment; your miracle-working mind and your positive new lifestyle are enough to do the job.

You are qualified to help yourself. Channel all the anger, guilt, and self-ridicule into constructive action. Draw upon your positive self-image, your confidence, your beliefs, and your accomplishments. It will soon be clear that the special person inside you has come out.

Today, look inside yourself and find a special person, one that is good, energetic, and achieving. Free that person.

*Today's Action Plan: I will take action to become who I really am. I will bring out my best.*

## December 12                          You're Not Alone

*To feel that one has a place in life solves half the problem of contentment.*
*—George E. Woodberry*

When you slip off your eating plan, you're not alone. When you feel like a miserable failure, you're not alone. When you're ready to give up on the whole world for good, you're not alone. Many others have felt that way.

When you get down on yourself, it's usually because you've drifted away from your three basic, simple needs: healthy eating, exercise, and a winning attitude. When you feel yourself getting troubled, check to see which need you've neglected and start satisfying it again.

Then, *talk* yourself out of your slump. Winners talk

out loud to themselves, telling themselves what they need to hear as no one else can. Finally, *work* yourself out of a slump. There is no substitute for taking action; it is the greatest motivator.

Everyone slips—you aren't alone. Today see that in order to win, you have to get into action each time you stumble.

*Today's Action Plan: I will understand that others have slipped too. Like them, I will get right up and continue.*

## December 13                    The Success in Rejection

*Few setbacks are as devastating as rejection.*
                        *—Dr. David Burns*

You phone a relative who is too busy to talk with you. A co-worker takes a coffee break without you. A sales clerk waits on a customer who arrives after you. You may regard such acts as rejection and proof of your unworthiness. But rejection can't exist unless you permit it.

The key to recovering from rejection is to use it as an occasion to reaffirm your value. That's not easy to do. Instead of affirming our self-worth, we often sabotage ourselves. We see rejection as proof that we are inept, unlovable, and unworthy of opportunity.

Stop taking rejection so seriously, exaggerating it, and beating yourself over the head with it. You deserve love and acceptance. Most of all, you deserve your own support. Achieving success means taking risks, and with risks, you may get some rejection. Every rejection is merely another chance to reaffirm yourself and thereby succeed.

Today, learn that you are the one who gives rejection

its capacity to hurt. Unless you assist it, it has no power of its own.

*Today's Action Plan: I will use rejection as a stepping stone to success, as a winner should.*

**December 14**                    **How Did It Feel to Be Fat?**

*It helps me to remember how miserable I was—the contrast is enough to make me want to maintain my weight loss.*

*—Diet group speaker*

Occasionally, recovering overeaters need to remember the negative feelings they once held about themselves. Once those feelings were impossible to confront; now it is a great relief to speak of them in the past tense.

What's it like to be fat? It's not being able to cross your legs. It's hating words like *plump, stout, chubby,* and *obese.* It's being out of breath. It's buttons straining and thighs chafing.

It's also covering your stomach when sitting, always pulling at clothes. It's feeling bloated and ugly. It's being embarrassed in public, never relaxed.

It's feeling ashamed, sick, guilty, and angry. It's feeling so worthless and beyond help that you eat even more.

Today, remember the misery of overeating, and take action to make new and wonderful memories for yourself.

*Today's Action Plan: I will remember the fat days so I know how far I've come. Today I will make thin memories.*

*One should . . . be able to see that things are hopeless
and yet be determined to make them otherwise.*
                                    —*F. Scott Fitzgerald*

Overeating created an underlying self-hate and
shame. Denial was the only way you could maintain a
shred of self-respect, so you concealed your weight with
loose clothing, you rationalized that everyone gained as
they aged, and you denied that you enjoyed sports or
dancing. Your clothes became larger and your breath
shorter. Finally, you were forced to face yourself, and
your denial mechanisms fell apart.

Resolve never to let your fat denial mechanisms work
again. Your life and your body are your top priorities.
Believe that you must take charge of food if you want
to do the things you denied yourself, if you want to live.

Make yourself the first priority in your life and you
will succeed. There's no other way.

Today, reject the fat denial mechanisms that only
served to delay really living your life.

*Today's Action Plan: I will base my daily life on my
action plan. I will never deny my top priority again.*

*An unexpected benefit of pain is the opportunity, even
the necessity, to be courageous.*

                                    —*Anonymous*

You can be an inspiration to your family, diet group,
and co-workers. As you lose weight, other people will
turn to you because they will see in you attitudes they
feel lacking in their own life.

Your three-part life plan is a creative living process

that makes you fascinating to other people. Think about it. In your re-creation process you heal your inner pain, restructure your self-image, and rebuild your body. All this takes courage, and courage is inspiring.

Your courage and your discipline will be a powerful inspiration to other people. You will have succeeded at a great task, a process others will want to copy.

Be a role model, but be aware of pitfalls. Don't begin to think that your success removes you from temptation. It doesn't. You must make your new lifestyle a life-long priority.

Today, you can be a source of inspiration for other people. Help them, but also resolve to keep your own program number one.

*Today's Action Plan: I will grow so that I can help others. I will inspire others, while reinforcing my own new life.*

## December 17                    Command Therapy

*The rhythm of life is intricate but orderly, tenacious but fragile. To keep that in mind is to hold the key to survival.*
                                   *—Shirley M. Hufstedler*

You need daily healing, because few things are as stressful as being overweight in a thin world. Controlling stress and tension is essential to taking charge of your health.

To be your own best healer, create a little inner refuge at stressful times of the day when you are prone to overeat. Relax and remember a feeling of happiness, then direct that feeling to the part of your body that needs it most.

You can go further yet with a technique called

"command therapy," which was originally designed to aid cancer patients. For overweight people, the method requires that you imagine bad fat cells being devoured by good thin cells. Imagine yourself healing by visualizing yourself thin. This technique has helped seriously ill people survive; why can't it help you? It's another way to take control of your body.

Today, focus your mind's healing power on your weight problem.

*Today's Action Plan: I will visualize thin cells attacking and replacing fat cells. I will be in charge of my own health.*

### December 18                          Take Today—All the Way

*I like to take this day—any day—and go to town with it.*

*—James Dickey*

This is a new day, a new challenge, and it begins for you with your next heartbeat. You have never lived this day before, never spoken, walked, laughed, or worked in this day. You're in charge of what you do with this day.

Use this day efficiently; use all of it to further your goals. Make time work for you today; allow it to become a self-valuing, productive experience. You need that and you deserve it too.

The first and greatest step today is to integrate all of your day into your healthy eating, exercise, and positive attitude program. It lights your day and prepares you to "go to town with it." You deserve a day like that.

See that today is fresh, waiting for you to make it a triumph.

*Today's Action Plan: I will make maximum use of today. I will integrate my three-part living program into the next twenty-four hours so that wonderful things become possible.*

**December 19**                                      **Rules of Self-Esteem**

*The noble soul has reverence for itself.*
                                        *—Friedrich Nietzsche*

Overeaters often treat themselves as bad children who need to be punished. This only smothers self-esteem. It's time to start treating yourself as an adult.

1. *Don't belittle yourself.* Constant negative messages like, "I can't do anything right," are untrue and unkind.

2. *Don't threaten yourself.* Warnings of "If you do that one more time, . . ." destroy self-esteem. You may have to make the same mistake again before you learn.

3. *Don't overprotect yourself.* When you always remove yourself from risk, you see yourself as someone who can't handle mistakes.

4. *Don't play hopscotch with your action plan.* When you train yourself to do something new, you must be consistent and systematic.

5. *Don't use guilt.* Thinking, "If I don't do that, I'm a rotten person" saps your energy.

Treat yourself in a calm, mature, self-respecting manner, just as you would treat any adult.

Today, see that punishing yourself only destroys self-esteem.

*Today's Action Plan: I will treat myself as an adult. I will not punish myself for mistakes, but will begin again.*

*Every individual has a place to fill in the world, and is important in some respect, whether he chooses to be so or not.*

*—Nathaniel Hawthorne*

If you really believe you are unique and have an independent worth, you'll be a winner. When things get tough, your absolute belief in your worth will keep you in action.

Uniqueness is not a guarantee of success, whether it's in losing weight or anything else, but it affirms that you can do for yourself what no one else can do.

You are unlimited. Never send negative messages to yourself; never affirm self-limitation. Affirm what you want to be. What you believe is what you are.

Today, face the wonderful fact of your uniqueness and see what its affirmation can mean in your life.

*Today's Action Plan: I will continue to develop a solid understanding of my unique worth. I will not limit, but affirm myself.*

*Happiness has many roots, but none more important than security.*

*—E. R. Stettinius Jr.*

Do you feel the need for some breathing space? Are family and friends filling your empty moments with their own priorities? Is your "to do" list at work or at home getting longer, not shorter? Are outside forces claiming precious spare moments?

If you feel you have little control over the direction of your day, take back control of your own time. It can be as simple as ensuring a few minutes to yourself or as major as emptying your appointment book for a day. Making your routine work better for you helps you feel in control and secure.

Being on your own side is simply a way to express self-consideration. You need that attitude to become a winner.

Today, take your own side. Whether you need empty spaces in your day or a sense that you are master of your own direction, take the necessary steps.

*Today's Action Plan: I will set priorities to include some empty space. I will arrange schedules that work best for me.*

### December 22                                     The Overdoer

*Untangling problems takes purpose, patience, and persistence.*

—*Frank Tyger*

Many overeaters are also overdoers, run ragged by superfull schedules and the sense that the whole world rests on their shoulders. To overdoers, every activity is a "should." If they don't do it, it won't get done.

Usually, this kind of overeater is really saying, "Don't look at my body, look at all the wonderful things I do," desperately needing to be admired. But how can such people be admired without killing themselves in the process?

Try to choose between the tasks you love and the extras that are "shoulds." You'll gain more time to devote to the jobs you decide to keep. Learn to admire yourself for your true value, not just as a workhorse.

Today, see that overdoing is another way to avoid responsibility for your overeating.

*Today's Action Plan: I will concentrate on certain important jobs and let the rest go. My primary responsibility is to control my overeating.*

## December 23 — Your Healing Mind

*The human mind can be trained to play an important part both in preventing disease and in overcoming it when it occurs.*

*—Norman Cousins*

The influence of mind on body was well known to ancient healers, yet scientific medicine focuses mostly on physical causes of illness—including overeating. The "cure" to being fat is thought to be a diet, but diet is only part of the answer.

Overeating can be influenced positively or negatively by your mental state. In other words, an event itself doesn't make you eat; it's how you react to it.

The brain overrides old thinking habits by introducing new habits that compete with and finally replace the old. If you formerly gave yourself failure messages, now give some positive ones. If you used to be out of control, now use self-management strategies to overwhelm the old helpless feelings. If your put healthy eating, exercise, and positive attitudes into your day, you will succeed.

Today, create attitudes of self-worth and control. Strong positive attitudes don't waste time dueling with old negative mind-sets—they overcome them.

*Today's Action Plan: I will follow a healing path. I will take good care of my mental state so my mind will take care of my body.*

*By the streets of "by and by," one arrives at the house of "never."*

— *Saavedra M. de Cervantes*

There is never a better time than today to build your own workable action plan. If you are waiting for just the right time, you'll wait forever.

All people are responsible for their own happiness. If you have a scapegoat for your overeating ("Dad always made me clean my plate"), you will only be momentarily comforted. If you carry a grudge against someone ("If she loved me enough, I wouldn't overeat"), it makes only you miserable, no one else.

The only life you can control is your own, and today is the only day you have to bring about meaningful changes in your life—not some future day.

You must be willing *today* to make the effort. Every day, you need to make an intelligent and mature decision to exchange the immediate gratification of overeating for a long-range, life-changing goal.

Today, accept full responsibility for your life. Say yes to maturity.

*Today's Action Plan: I will make a lifesaving decision to take charge of my recovery. I will be responsible for all that I do today.*

*There can be no peace of mind without strength of mind.*

— *Eric B. Gutkind*

For almost a year you have been working on your mental fitness. Today you are stronger than ever; you have declared peace within yourself. Once you were in conflict, it seemed, with the very air you breathed. The imbalance between what you wanted and what you were actually doing created an unbearable disharmony.

When you do what you know you need to do, peace of mind envelops you. Peace, not food, becomes your element. You allow nothing and no one to disturb this peace.

Above all, keep your mind in a state of calm. You have learned to let go of distrust, fear, and self-blame. You have willed your negative self-critic to be silent and have filled your mind to the brim with joy and peace.

You are truly in charge of your peace. Keep it with you always.

Today, you are your own peacemaker. You are the creative decision-maker of your life. You are the director of your energy.

*Today's Action Plan: I will make my mind strong so that I can establish peace within myself. Peace of mind comes through action.*

### December 26    Beating the Fear of Expectation

*I was not prepared to be thin. I was like the poor girl who suddenly gets rich. How was I supposed to act?*
*—A successful dieter*

Reaching your natural weight, the one most comfortable for you, is a moment of supreme joy, one of the happiest in your life, and it should be. It took incredible courage and persistence.

When you began your program, you went through a transformation. It was exciting and people praised you along the way. But now you are no longer the dieter who needs special consideration. Now you are expected to perform at home, on the job, and at social occasions.

People may say, "You look wonderful. You don't need to take all these precautions anymore." Don't you believe it! You must keep doing all those things that got you to this day. Carry on with your good eating management to stabilize and maintain your weight. Continue your physical fitness routine. Practice your action plan principles. Persevere and stay healthy.

Today, whip any fear by continuing all those things that made you a winner. Enjoy your new life.

*Today's Action Plan: I will take charge of weight stabilization. I will continue to use positive attitudes.*

## December 27

### Diet without Exercise Is No Diet at All

*The bathroom scale tells you you're doing something right, but you actually haven't improved your body composition.*
—*Donald Layman*

The nutritionist quoted above conducted an interesting experiment on a group of obese rats. They starved off 75 percent of their body weight, yet maintained the same proportion of fat. And worse, if they regained their weight, the proportion of body fat increased even more. The same phenomenon applies to people who diet but don't exercise.

The answer lies in healthy eating plus exercise. On this kind of schedule, your energized body gets into the habit of burning off fat. When you reach your maintenance weight, you may actually need to eat more just to keep your weight from going too low!

To maintain your natural weight, keep a balance between food intake and energy outgo. To win, all you need is the commitment.

Diet with exercise is a winning proposition. Today, commit yourself to action on every front.

*Today's Action Plan: I will think of exercise as the game that destroys fat forever. I will put myself in control of my life and never let go.*

### December 28                What Would You Wish?

*For of all sad words of tongue or pen,*
*The saddest are these: "It might have been!"*
                    —*John Greenleaf Whittier*

Right now, do you have everything you want from life? Probably not, but you can feel happy knowing you're heading in the right direction.

Many people who have lived a full life span don't regret what they have done as much as what they haven't done. Pretend you are eighty and lamenting your failure to reach a certain goal. Did being overweight prevent you from achieving your desire?

It might have been that, in pursuing a career of achievement, your work also took on a purpose. What you did for a living became meaningful in a way you hadn't expected.

It might have been that you constantly lamented life's unfairness. Life might have been good and joyous, but you did not rescue the joy from the trap of emotional pain.

It might have been that life gave you a chance to be what you could have been, experience what you could have experienced, and love what you could have loved. What did you do with that chance?

Someday will you look back and say sadly, "It might have been"? Or will you say with satisfaction, "It was"? It's your choice.

Today, determine that you will experience all this day has to offer.

*Today's Action Plan: I will work to realize my ambition. I will not take refuge from problems in overeating.*

## December 29          What Do You Have to Live For?

*I believe that only one person in a thousand knows the trick of really living in the present.*

—Storm Jameson

Every minute of the day is an unrepeatable miracle for us to use. Let's use these small miracles to strengthen our attitudes toward ourselves and our place in the world.

Today is yours for action and imagination. Taking charge of your life is an act of imagination. It is a search through your desires, a lifelong discovery process.

In time-lapse photography, a rose gradually unfolds one petal at a time until it has created its own full-blown, openhearted beauty. Each minute of today is like that rose petal. As your day unfolds, you create a harmonious, beautiful life, free forever of the pain of overeating.

Use every minute of today to take practical action for weight control and to search for the desires that power your determination.

*Today's Action Plan: I will bloom, using the action process of living in the present. I will give myself all the time I need to discover the beauty within me.*

*Have you learned lessons only of those who admired you, and were tender with you, and stood aside for you? Have you not learned great lessons from those who rejected you, and braced themselves against you, or disputed the passage with you?*

—*Walt Whitman*

We've all stumbled at times, but here you are, marching ahead, risking, and learning—even from those who don't accept you. Such courage as yours is the basis of security, self-value, and ability to achieve. You refuse to be handicapped by a food pacifier.

Think of yourself as a winner when you function in a crisis without overeating.

Think of yourself as a winner when you truly believe that people love and value you just as you are—and you do too.

Think of yourself as a winner when you risk your feelings to accomplish what you know needs to be done.

Think of yourself as a winner when you practice your new action plan.

Today, learn from others, but receive your sense of meaning from within. You have a purpose and goals.

*Today's Action Plan: I will think of myself as one who no longer needs a food pacifier. I am a winner.*

*Keep going, don't quit. Imagine. Scrutinize.*
*Once more with feeling: think.*

—*James McConkey*

There is no last word to this book. The story doesn't end; it just keeps beginning again. Each time it begins, each time you plant positive thoughts in your mind or take charge of your eating, you become more independent. You deserve to grasp so much more of life.

Some days it seems as if your positive thoughts refuse to take root. Believe that they will. Change is hard, but you can do it. Change is the root of all achievement.

Together we have come to the end of your beginning. Many messages have been sent to you through these pages. Next year, changed as you are from the journey, new messages will be waiting here for you.

It has been a long trip, but one well worth taking.

Today, renew your commitment to healthy eating and physical and mental fitness. You have made yourself a winner.

*Today's Action Plan: I will realize that today is as much of a challenge and opportunity as the first day of the year. I will commit myself anew to uncovering my essential self.*

# Resources

## Cookbooks

American Heart Association. *American Heart Association Cookbook.* 5th ed. New York: Random House, 1991.

Baird, Pat. *Pyramid Cookbook: Pleasure of the Food Guide Pyramid.* New York: Henry Holt and Co., 1993.

Brody, Jane. *Jane Brody's Good Food Book: Living the High Carbohydrate Way.* New York: Norton, 1985.

Hughes, Nancy S. *Four-Course, Four-Hundred Calorie Meal Cookbook: Quick and Easy Recipes for Delicious Low-Calorie, Low-Fat Dinners.* Chicago: Contemporary Books, 1991.

Shulman, Martha Rose. *Mediterranean Light: Delicious Recipes from the World's Healthiest Cuisine.* New York: Bantam, 1989.

Woodruff, R. D. Sandra. *Secrets of Fat-Free Baking.* Garden City Park, N.Y.: Avery Publishing Group, 1995.

## Exercise

Getchell, Bud. *The Fitness Book.* Indianapolis, Ind.: Benchmark Press, 1987.

Liptak, Karen. *Fitness for Women.* New York: Gallery Books, 1990.

*Walking* magazine, 9-11 Harcourt Street, Boston, MA 92116. 1-800-678-0881.

White, Timothy P., and the editors of University of California at Berkeley Wellness Letter. *The Wellness Guide to Lifelong Fitness.* New York: Rebus, 1993.

## Fat Counters

Bellerson, Karen J. *The Complete Up-to-Date Fat Book: A Guide to Fat, Calories, and Fat Percentages in Your Food.* 2nd ed. Garden City Park, N.Y.: Avery Publishing Group, 1993.

Fit Choice 1-800-790-1994

A magnetized plastic sheet showing fat grams of hundreds of common foods and placing the foods in the appropriate section of the U.S. Agriculture Department's Food Pyramid.

## Nutrition

Blonz, Edward R. *Your Personal Nutritionist: Fiber and Fat Counter.* New York: Signet, 1995.

*Eating Well* magazine. Telemedia Communications, Inc. Ferry Road, Charlotte, VT 95545.

Kirschmann, John D. *Nutritional Almanac.* 3d ed. New York: McGraw Hill, 1990.

*Vegetarian Times* magazine. P.O. Box 570, Oak Park, IL 60303.

## Positive Living

Chopra, Deepak, M.D. *Perfect Health.* New York: Harmony Books, 1991.

DeAngelis, Barbara. *Real Moments.* New York: Delacorte Press, 1994.

Mason, L. John. *Guide to Stress Reduction.* Berkeley: And Or Press, 1981

Null, Gary. *Change Your Life Now: Get Out of Your Head, Get Into Your Life.* Deerfield Beach, Fla.: Health Communications, 1993.

## Self-Esteem

Branden, Nathaniel. *How to Raise Your Self-Esteem.* New York: Bantam Books, 1988.

Rodin, Judith. *Body Traps.* New York: William Morrow, 1992.

Sanford, Linda Tscherhart, and Mary Ellen Donovan. *Women and Self-Esteem.* New York: Viking Penguin, 1985.

## Size-Acceptance
National Association to Advance Fat Acceptance, P.O. Box 188620, Sacramento, CA 95818, 1-800-442-1214.

## Starch-Centered Vegetarian Diet
McDougall, John A., M.D. *The McDougall Program for Maximum Weight Loss.* New York: Dutton, 1994.

Ornish, Dean, M.D. *Eat More, Weigh Less: Dr. Dean Ornish's Life Choice Program for Losing Weight Safely While Eating Abundantly.* New York: HarperCollins, 1993.

## 25-fat Gram Diet Plan
Page, Helen Cassidy, John Speer Schroeder, M.D., and Tara Coghlin Dickson. *The Stanford Life Plan for a Healthy Heart.* San Francisco: Chronicle Books, 1996.

## Weight Maintenance
Brownell, Kelly D., and Judith Rodin. *The Weight Maintenance Survival Guide.* Dallas: American Health Publishing Co., 1990.

## What Mother Nature Did to Us
Beller, Anne Scott. *Fat and Thin: A Natural History of Obesity.* New York: Farrar, Straus and Giroux, 1977.

# Index

# Index

## About the Author

Jeane Eddy Westin is an author, teacher, and consultant. Her published works include *The Thin Book, The Thin Book 2*, and *Breaking Out of Your Fat Cell*. She has also written more than 250 articles published in numerous national publications, including *Ms., Woman's Day, Parade*, and *Weight Watchers*.

*Other titles that will interest you . . .*

**Fat is a Family Affair**
A Guide for People with Eating Disorders and Those Who Love
Them
  *by Judi Hollis, Ph.D.*
National eating disorders expert Judi Hollis shows how the
Twelve Steps can be used to solve the relationship problems of
compulsive overeaters. Judi's own success story, and those of
others told in this book, help you redefine and improve your
relationships. 171 pp.
Order No. 1091

**Food for Thought**
Daily meditations for eating disorder sufferers by someone who
shares the pain and joys. Written in the tradition of *Twenty-Four
Hours a Day,* this daily meditation book is used by members of
Overeaters Anonymous and weight loss groups. 400 pp.
Order No. 1074

**Codependent No More**
How to Stop Controlling Others and Start Caring for Yourself
  *by Melody Beattie*
A healing touchstone for readers struggling to detach from
intense concern and care for others, this book provides healthy
suggestions on how to begin caring for yourself. Best-selling
author Melody Beattie addresses topics such as dealing with
anger, removing the victim, learning the art of acceptance, setting goals, and living our own life. 208 pp.

**▧HAZELDEN**®
**For price and order information, or a free catalog, please call
our Telephone Representatives.**
1-800-328-9000 (Toll-Free U.S., Canada, and the Virgin Islands)
1-612-257-4010 (Outside the U.S. and Canada)
1-612-257-1331 (24-Hour FAX)
http://www.Hazelden.org. (World Wide Web Site on the Internet)
Pleasant Valley Road • P.O. Box 176
Center City, MN 55012-0176